'This book is a substantial addition to importance of the natural environment offers a variety of fascinating and though different cultural and individual perceptions of nature and the outside world. With increasing realisation that it is possible to live well with dementia, this collection of papers should be essential reading on a vital but unexplored aspect of person-centred care.'

— Richard Humphries, Assistant Director
(Policy), The King's Fund, London

'Marshall and Gilliard challenge us to think beyond the threshold of the care home and what are all too often poorly utilised token corners of green. They address the consequences of being contained, constrained and chemically controlled, but at its heart is a demand to think big, listen and support people with dementia to benefit from getting outside; is that too much to ask?'

— Colm Cunningham, Visiting Professor at the University of Salford
and Director, HammondCare Dementia Centre, Australia

'This wonderful book made my heart sing – a powerful exploration of the rich diversity of our lived experience of the outside world, the connection between mother nature and human nature and our collective need for breathing spaces that we recognise, that can bring a deep sense of familiarity, that let us know we are valid, that our place in a world we recognise is intact. Read this book and be inspired to connect people with dementia to outdoor spaces that will resonate with them – this will change their lives and bring them moments of peace, clarity and well-being.'

— Andy Bradley, Founding Director, Frameworks 4 Change

*Creating Culturally Appropriate Outside Spaces
and Experiences for People with Dementia*

Creating
Culturally
Appropriate
Outside Spaces
and
Experiences
for People with
Dementia

Using Nature and the Outdoors in Person-Centred Care

Edited by Mary Marshall and Jane Gilliard

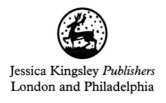

Jessica Kingsley *Publishers*
London and Philadelphia

Figure 5.4 (page 77) reproduced with permission from The King's Fund, London.

First published in 2014
by Jessica Kingsley Publishers
73 Collier Street
London N1 9BE, UK
and
400 Market Street, Suite 400
Philadelphia, PA 19106, USA

www.jkp.com

Library of Congress Cataloging in Publication Data
A CIP catalog record for this book is available from the Library of Congress

British Library Cataloguing in Publication Data
A CIP catalogue record for this book is available from the British Library

ISBN 978 1 84905 514 7
eISBN 978 0 85700 927 2

Printed and bound in Great Britain

Contents

Acknowledgements

Grateful thanks to Dr Jamal Hilal, an old-age psychiatrist at St George's Park Hospital for the Northumberland, Tyne and Wear, NHS Foundation Mental Health Trust, whose reflections we used to illustrate the Introduction. He was born and lived in the Sudan until the early 1990s and returns regularly to visit his family and contribute to teaching programmes. He has worked in different parts of his country, Sudan, including the southern region, which is a separate country now.

Wendy Hulko would like to acknowledge the Secwepemc Nation and colleagues from Interior Health (IH) and Thompson Rivers University (TRU) for collaborating on the programme of research, particularly Danielle Wilson and Brad Anderson of Aboriginal Health, Elisabeth Antifeau of IH, and Star Mahara of TRU Nursing. A special thank you to Jennifer Mackie for commenting on an earlier draft of Wendy's chapter. Funding for the work came from the Interior Health Authority, Michael Smith Foundation for Health Research, Canadian Dementia Knowledge Translation Network, Alzheimer Society of Canada, and Canadian Institutes of Health Research.

Introduction

Why Do We Need to Understand Cultural Differences?

MARY MARSHALL AND JANE GILLIARD

Dementia and the diversity of life experience

Every human being needs to get outside. They need to have contact with nature. This seems so obvious that it is surprising that it needs to be said. It is true of all of us. Sadly, people with dementia, especially if they are in a care home or hospital (see Care Commission and Mental Welfare Commission 2009, for example), are often deprived of contact with nature. There may be many reasons such as access issues (the person with dementia may live upstairs or the door to the outside may be locked); the staff may have neither the knowledge of the importance of being outside nor the time to ensure that going out happens; or management policies may not emphasise contact with nature. The weather is constantly given as a reason: it may rain, it is raining, it has rained or it is too cold or too hot or too windy. Yet weather is part of nature and part of the experience of being outside.

This book is about a fifth reason which is, as far as we know, neglected. This is that the outside space provided may be unfamiliar, strange, unacceptable or perhaps even frightening in some way. It seems to us that we need to consider what was most familiar to people with dementia from their youth and to use this knowledge to ensure that the outside spaces and the activities there make sense to each person and that they are comfortable with them.

In this book we look at familiar outside spaces for many different cultures and geographical locations. This introduction will be illustrated with some observations by Dr Jamal Hilal, an old-age psychiatrist who came to the UK from Sudan. He offered us some reflections after a visit to his family in Sudan. We have used his reflections here since the landscapes he describes are very different indeed from those of rich, industrialised countries. We are both British and we wanted to use these reflections to remind us that some people who live and work in the UK have extraordinarily different views of what is familiar in nature.

We know that people working with people with dementia may never work with people from the cultures and places described in our book, but we are keen to make a point about differences and the need to be sensitive to the backgrounds of people with dementia who may be unable to share with us what would be most familiar to them and would bring them most comfort. A key point we will return to is the need to understand the detail of the differences; one urban location is not the same as another, one African country is not the same as another, and so on. Jamal Hilal makes this point when he describes the two different kinds of worlds within Sudan:

> The people of my country in so many areas are nomadic shepherds and hunters/gatherers until this day. They live around a herd of beasts of burden and stock with limited agricultural experiments that can afford to be shut down swiftly in the haste of moving to the next stop of survival and relative prosperity. In contrast, some of the Nilotic communities in the north of the country have long ago established agricultural practices in that narrow region by the banks of the River Nile with the focus being the crops and produce, and hence is the limited development of the industry. With a closer look at the city dwellers in Sudan, one can still see the features of the wandering nomadic lifestyle which is much deeper than how some places might look in terms of landscape and agriculture.

Mental and physical needs that can be met by going outside

First, though, we think it may be helpful to spell out why people need to get outside. Sometimes the case needs to be made on mental and physical health grounds, which predominate in our list. We then provide, as this introduction progresses, a whole set of other more subtle, but no less important, reasons.

Our initial list is as follows:

1. Vitamin D is important for bone and muscle strength. Given the catastrophic consequences of a fall for people with dementia, this should have a high priority. For sufficient vitamin D for health, the arms and face need to be exposed to direct sun for ten minutes each day between April and October (McNair *et al.* 2013).

2. Circadian rhythm, or the body clock as it is sometimes known, is often disrupted in people with dementia. It can cause them and those caring for them a great many problems. A simple way to rectify this for many people with dementia is exposure to morning light and darkness at night (McNair *et al.* 2013).

3. Seasonal affective disorder (SAD) results in apathy and low mood, which is not helpful if you are coping with dementia. Light is again the way to help (McNair *et al.* 2013).

4. Exercise has been found in many studies (e.g. Larson *et al.* 2006) to prevent dementia and to help those who already have it. Exercise is easy and enjoyable outside where it may be unsatisfying inside.

5. Diminished lung capacity and diseases such as COPD (chronic obstructive pulmonary disease) and asthma are common in older people, yet not getting enough oxygen into your lungs can affect concentration in people with dementia. The air is usually better outside.

6. There are many activities which can take place outside in a very straightforward way, and since activities are the key dementia 'treatment', then getting outside is clearly beneficial.

7. Many of today's very old people spent a lot of their lives outside since they did not have cars and they often worked outside too. For them it is normal to be outside some of the time. Past interests can be stimulated by outside objects and activities. It can also reinforce or lead to rediscovery of a past interest.

8. Your identity can change outside. People with dementia are recipients of social and health care in care homes and hospitals, yet when they are outside they can be themselves.

9. People with dementia with the normal hearing impairments of later life can find noise inside very overwhelming. Outside is often quieter and calmer.

10. People who are dying seem to need contact with nature very intensely – we will return to this need later.

Diverse childhood memories

Our book is based on the assumption that familiar outside spaces are those we knew as children and that these are the ones that will make sense to a person with dementia. It is obvious, when you watch children, that contact with nature has a profound intensity. If we asked you for your most vivid childhood memory of being outside, what would you reply? Jane would say seaside and Mary would say oak woods. Since these memories are also likely to be the most familiar if, and when, we get dementia, then seeing them outside or being taken to them will encourage us to go out and relish them. It is therefore beholden on those of us who want to encourage people with dementia to go outside for all the important mental and physical health reasons to provide external spaces and experiences that resonate with people's pasts.

This is not a straightforward objective. In the 2011 census 13 per cent (7.5 million) of the residents of England and Wales were born outside the UK. We may be in a place with different geography, climate, beliefs and traditions from those we know best. There is also migration within countries. In the last century the enormous growth of the greater Tokyo metropolitan area to more than 35 million people was mainly a result of rural-to-urban migration, and the same is true of Mumbai in the 21st century. In the UK the towns surrounding London, such as Swindon and Milton Keynes, are the fastest-growing urban areas in Europe, with the result that a lot of people will age in a different place from where they grew up. Thus, being far from what is most familiar is not just a result of migration from one country to another.

In these times of unprecedented urbanisation and migration, many people live very far from the place where they were children. Even if we are in the same country, children born in rural areas of mountains, seaside or meadows may now live in towns. Jane's mother was born in rural Kent and she now lives in a small village. Her delight as a child was birds and she has been able to continue to enjoy this throughout her life as long as she lives at home. Mary's father was born and raised in India and as a child went to Ooty (Ootacamund, the Queen of Hill Stations in the Nilgiri Hills) when it was hot in the cities. He too was luckily able to enjoy a familiar landscape of trees, a loch and hills from his garden in Scotland when he got dementia.

Being alert to cultural differences within the population of people with dementia is stressed in numerous British policy documents. *Living Well with Dementia* stresses the importance of 'working across diverse populations affected by dementia, e.g. different language groups, minority ethnic groups' (Department of Health 2009, p.39). The Foreword of the first Scottish Dementia Strategy (2010–2013) mentions: 'We must ensure that the needs of minority groups such as BSL [British Sign Language] users and people from diverse ethnic groups are not missed' (Scottish Government 2011). The National Dementia Vision for Wales says: 'We need to plan services to take into account the needs of people who live in rural and urban settings and ensure that language and cultural needs and preferences are catered for' (Welsh Assembly Government and Alzheimer's Society 2011). Our book takes these important objectives and asserts that they are important for the design and use of outside spaces as well as all other aspects of dementia care.

Not just gardens

At this point we want to be clear that we are not only talking about gardens; our use of the term 'outside spaces' is deliberate. Gardens are, by definition, 'an area of land usually planted with grass, trees, flower beds etc. adjoining a house' (Collins Dictionary 1987), although the term may mean different things in different languages and cultures. Jamal Hilal's observation is:

> The garden is a vague entity in the Sudanese language. The Arabic term is 'Jinaina', which means 'a miniature of paradise',

proposing a multitude of colour, fragrance and leisure to the senses and mind, but in the Sudanese context it is used loosely to describe the greenery which is rich in shade and coolness. This can be an area of turf with different scattered bushes and some flowers, the most popular of which are the sunflower and the bougainvillea; both are low-maintenance plants that require little care once grown deep enough to fend for themselves. The word 'Jinaina' can also be used to mean a plantation of fruit-bearing trees such as mangoes, oranges, limes and the like. The emphasis remains on the shady and cool atmosphere that makes the heat less ruthless on the bodies and minds.

Many people's most vivid memories of outside and nature are not gardens at all. If this book achieves nothing else, we hope that this understanding will remain with our readers. Too many places that do make great efforts with their outside spaces provide a 'sensory garden' – a garden with traditional fragrant bushes and flowers. Whereas this may make perfect sense to people who have always lived in a spacious town or suburb where each house has a garden, this is not the majority even in the UK. We would encourage people who want to create outside spaces that are familiar to a diverse group of people with dementia to think in terms of 'outside rooms' or several different spaces for people of different backgrounds.

Of course, the contact people with dementia have with outside and nature need not be limited to the area adjacent to the house, as Neil Mapes' chapter demonstrates. He also shows us that people with dementia can enjoy new experiences of nature, and we are keen to support these very special initiatives. However, our main concern is that people with dementia living in hospitals and care homes rarely go outside, and the unfamiliarity of the outside spaces may be a contributory factor.

Jamal Hilal told us that the conventional British garden might be too much for an elderly Sudanese person with dementia:

The harsh heat, the endless dust and the pursuit of survival rather than leisure are very strong elements in shaping the mind frame about gardens and gardening, so how would that mind frame be when it is afflicted by a degeneration of its faculties and functions? How would a person from this background respond to suddenly being in a place of full colour and fragrance? Mind you, the majority are believers in the afterlife, which should be, they hope, in Paradise, that is 'Janna' in Arabic, the original bigger version of Jinaina. The carnival of colour might be too much and confusing, or the person might believe they are no longer in this life, that they have died and that they are entitled to the complementary rewards of being in Janna.

Our chapters

At this point we want to introduce our contributors and why we think their individual chapters have important lessons for us in our efforts to provide experiences of nature that are familiar and meaningful. We have organised our presentations with subheadings of key issues that we think make the chapter especially significant, although there are of course overlaps between the chapters.

The knowledge and contribution of carers

We wanted to start this book with a chapter from a relative, and Beth Britton provides a very moving account of her father, a farmer, and how care homes deprived him of contact with what was most important to him. Most care homes would be challenged by this, although there are some amazing exceptions such as Neville Williams House in Birmingham where they have chickens, pigs, goats and rabbits for the residents to tend and relate to (Gilliard and Marshall 2012). If there was a greater understanding from staff about the importance of nature to people with dementia, they would find ways of sustaining this link. We hope our book stimulates a greater understanding. Beth Britton encapsulates what this book is about when she says:

> That type of natural environment was always my father's real home. It was a place where his human spirit connected with the universe in a way that was timeless. It was something he would have strived to protect and defend before his dementia developed, and something that he needed to be kept in touch with during his time in care. In a communal setting there are so many different interpretations of what makes an outdoor space

something that is reminiscent of the residents' former lives – from people who grew up playing on perfectly manicured lawns surrounded by topiary, to people like my father, who embraced the natural world and all its irregularities.

The seasons

Our next chapter is about Japan, a very different culture from any in the UK. We invited Yutaka Inoue to contribute because we were keen to provide a complete contrast – to make the point about diversity. We also knew that nature is very important to Japanese people. We learn from his chapter that the seasons are highly significant; for example, cherry blossom time. We know in the UK that one reason for going outside and seeing nature is that it orientates people with dementia to the seasons. In the UK, for example, our spirits rise as we see blossom after the winter. Judith Jones makes this point very movingly in her chapter. Thus it is not just the outside space that is important – but the opportunity to be exposed to the seasons in all their manifestations. Jamal Hilal says of Sudan:

> Abundance of sand and endless dusty ground is almost all what you see flying low into Sudan from the north border. Save the River Nile, marching slowly across the desert and the poor savannah. The first moments off the aeroplane are like a new birth; the first breath is harsh and rather painfully dry. This is the usual welcome of Khartoum, which can be much milder in the winter months from November to about the end of March. The peak of the heat in May to July is one of the yearly ordeals endured by the people of the central and northern parts of Sudan. When it goes up to fifty degrees Celsius you can hardly see real people, rather their ghosts and dormant inner beings. This can be true for most parts of the country, but the worst in summer is the coast of the Red Sea, being saturated with humidity on top of the scalding heat.

For Sidsel Bjørneby, Beth Britton and Gillean Maclean, our contributors who are talking about people reared in rural areas, there is a particularly strong link with the seasons. In Norway they would have triggered a migration to and from the higher pastures in some communities and from the cities to the summer cottages.

Dementia, nature and poetry

The chapter about Japan also makes the link between dementia and poetry; a connection reinforced by our inclusion of two poems by people with dementia from collections by John Killick (2008, 2010). This link between poetry and nature is a deep recurring one which is outside the focus of this book, but we would like to make the point here that the link between dementia and nature is connected to all aspects of dementia care, including the arts. Patrick Brenchley has mixed feelings about the Aran islands but he is clear that:

> Up to a point
> but not all of the time
> the scenes come back to me
> strongly and with great pleasure.

Yutaka Inoue also makes the point about nature and poetry, describing a woman who gained huge benefit from composing poetry about nature – in this case a tanka, which is a poem with 31 syllables:

> Looking up at sky
> without a cloud,
> I longed for
> my old home on the coast
> with a view of azure ocean.

Activity and nature

Neil Mapes' chapter presents contact with nature as enjoyment, entertainment and relaxation. Sometimes this is tailored to people's interests and sometimes it is something completely new, such as sailing. We should never assume that people with dementia do not continue to enjoy new experiences. He is clear that being active outside shows 'how we can maintain our personal and emotional connection with nature, despite having dementia'. Both Judith Jones and Yutaka Inoue emphasise the potential of outside for activities which we listed at the start as a crucial 'treatment' for dementia. Sharing and enjoying activities together is part of life itself. For us, Neil Mapes is fundamentally talking about British experiences of nature. For most British people, the park is their most familiar outside space, a point made too by Karen Franks and Kate Andrews

Woods and the seaside are also part of what it is to be British. We can contrast this with the chapter about Japan where the key cultural aspects of nature are cherry blossom and autumn colours.

Staff as well as people with dementia

The attitudes and experiences of nature of the staff of any facility (or indeed visiting at home) will have a big impact on the person with dementia, since they will encourage or neglect contact with nature in their care. The chapter by Margaret-Anne Tibbs raises this issue by sharing the attitudes and experiences of some southern African staff and some southern African friends. Urbanisation is a big issue throughout Africa and many people live far away from their roots.

Being outside is normal for many people, especially those who come from rural areas, as several of our chapters demonstrate. We need to understand that it may be a deep craving for some older people and they suffer when denied it, as Beth Britton so clearly shows in the story of her father.

A link with the past, a sense of continuity

Margaret-Anne Tibbs makes a key point about the desire of older people to return to the familiar place of their birth and upbringing, and for many this is about a rural area. We know the imaginative use of iPads to bring up photographs of places where people were born or reared (Lloyd-Yeates 2013) and the enormous pleasure this can give to someone with dementia, as can old photographs. Reminiscence is a well-established tool for dementia care (see Gibson 2011, for example), but more could be done to emphasise outside spaces and nature as a trigger. For people who have neither iPads nor photographs, actually going there is the only chance they will get to restore the links with their distant past. The language in some cultures such as rural southern Africa and the First Nation Canadians in Wendy Hulko's chapter is about 'ancestors'. Although many of us would not use these terms, the link with childhood can provide a sense of continuity for those we are caring for – it completes the circle of life, in a sense. This must be especially important for those approaching death, and we should never assume that people with dementia are any different from anyone else in this respect.

The challenge of the hospital setting

We asked Sarah Waller and Abigail Masterson to write us a chapter because we are very well aware of the serious challenges of providing contact with nature for people in hospital. Given that about 25 per cent of people in any acute hospital (Sampson *et al.* 2009) have dementia, this is a challenge that cannot be neglected in a book like this. In one sense this is a chapter about a culture of care rather than a culture of the patient.

Concern about patients with dementia has led to it being a priority in the English and new Scottish dementia strategies. As the Department of Health (2010) document *Quality Outcomes for People with Dementia* points out: '40% of people in hospital have dementia; the excess cost is estimated to be £6m per annum in the average General Hospital; co-morbidity with general medical conditions is high, people with dementia stay longer in hospital' (this figure relates to all hospitals, not just general hospitals).

Along with the obvious challenges of the acute sector, such as rapid through-put, very active treatment and a pre-occupation with infection control, there is the fact that most acute beds are above the ground floor. This should not be a barrier, but hospitals are no longer built with balconies and verandas, so it is a challenge which has to be met by art, light and views. It has long been known (Ulrich 2001) that views of nature speed up the healing process, but this well-established fact is often ignored by hospital designers and builders.

The importance of nature at the end of life

This issue was in our list of the well-established benefits of outside to people with dementia, and it is obviously especially important in the hospital setting. Sarah Waller and Abigail Masterson stress this from their project:

> Furthermore, consultations undertaken as part of a phase of the EHE programme particularly focused on improving environments for palliative care patients consistently showed that links to nature and the natural world were extremely important for people at the end of their lives and their visitors. Views of nature and/or being able to go outside were highly valued, as were the use of natural materials and the incorporation of the

elements, internal planting and the use of artworks depicting nature in interior designs.

The detail of past experience is crucial

Sidsel Bjørneby, at our request, has written about the Scandinavian tradition of summer cottages, but she includes the range of backgrounds of people in Norway who were reared in rural areas. They can be mountain people, seafarers or farmers. Furthermore, she introduces a new concept – that of seasonal migration both within rural areas and from city to country in the summer. Her chapter emphasises that you have to know the detail of people's past experiences in order to provide a familiar outside space or outside activities. This diversity of rural experiences is also in Beth Britton's story of her father, and Gillean Maclean's stories of different people in rural and island communities in Scotland. Sidsel Bjørneby's final paragraph brings a lot of themes together:

> Nature itself is sufficient as entertainment – birds singing, mountain streams, the smell of fresh air or the sound and smell of the sea, maybe a taste of wild berries; these are all sensory elements of value and provide a basis for actively bringing out memories and talking about them.

Even in rural areas, relating to the outside is not easy

We asked Gillean Maclean to write us a chapter about rural and island communities since she has always worked in these communities as a Church of Scotland minister and her mother was in a care home in her parish until she died. A substantial minority of people still live in the country in the UK and you could assume that contact with nature would be obvious for rural people in care homes and hospitals in rural areas. However, the fact is that most care homes and hospitals are in urban areas and are often away from the places from which people were admitted. Even for establishments that are in rural areas, staff have to have the time and often the transport to take people to places that are familiar. Yet the people with dementia Gillean Maclean spoke to were quite clear that they would really suffer if they lived away from views that were important to them, such as the sea or fields. The

English Dementia Strategy *Living Well with Dementia* (Department of Health 2009) specifically mentions rural and island communities:

> It should take account of the fact that the needs of some groups (e.g. those with a learning disability and dementia, younger people with dementia, those from minority ethnic groups, or those from rural, island or traveller communities) may be different from those of the majority population, and may require specifically tailored approaches.

Attitudes to nature can be part of deeply held belief systems

We asked both Wendy Hulko and Joan Domicelj to contribute because they both know a lot about very ancient peoples – Wendy as a researcher and Joan as a conservationist. We know that these cultures have a deep understanding of nature and that humans are part of it, not separate from it. The settings of Western Canada and rural Australia are very different, but the beliefs are similar at a fundamental level.

We all need to make sense of our lives by imposing our own personal or cultural meanings on our experiences. For the Secwepemc people of Western Canada, even dementia has a meaning. The Elders see the causes as largely social and environmental, resulting from factors such as dietary changes, chemical medications, pollution, etc. However, the linking factor between these two chapters is encapsulated in Wendy's sentence:

> The idea that Indigenous people honour the land and all of the creatures who inhabit it and recognize this interconnectedness is grounded in reality – past and contemporary.

This honouring of the land and interconnectedness links, to different degrees, all our contributors, but it is most clearly expressed by these ancient cultures.

It is not just what nature looks like but what you do in it

Almost all of our contributors suggest ways of interacting with nature; at its crudest this is about activities, but it is also about long-held traditions and ways of life. Sidsel Bjørneby points out how hard it is for urban, younger staff to understand what would be familiar to the people with dementia in their charge. Beth Britton talks about the failure of people looking after her father to understand that he needed to see farms and farm animals. Wendy's suggestions include:

> Building on nature-assisted therapy in dementia care by introducing more culturally relevant programming such as berry-picking, fishing, and gathering medicines as well as bringing the outdoors inside through activities such as canning salmon would be well received by First Nation Elders.

The importance of the philosophy of the care home

Judith Jones was asked to contribute because we knew that anthroposophy had a strong belief in nature not unlike that of Indigenous people. She says:

> Our health and wellbeing depends on a balanced relationship of body, soul and spirit which we see being thrown into imbalance in dementia. In Steiner's view, illness manifests itself primarily in body and soul while the spirit remains intact. It follows that for the person with dementia the spiritual need for recognition, respect and dignity does not change. Likewise, opportunities to experience beauty, rhythm and meaningful activity may contribute to letting spiritual integrity shine through the illness.

Her descriptions of what happens in her care home, based on the Steiner principles, puts most care homes to shame. She shows how nature can be part of everyday life – not just through a garden but by using every aspect of nature: the stars, food, seasons. We need this approach to be part of the philosophy of any care setting to enrich what is often a much-diminished life for people with dementia. Nature is all around us – we just have to interact with it. As one of her carers says:

> Nature has no boundaries. In its global and generous way it welcomes everyone, never judging anyone's behaviour, like a mother waiting for her child to come home after a long, long journey.

People who have always lived in cities have
varied and unexpected links to nature

Karen Franks and Kate Andrews offered to write us a chapter when we met Karen Franks at a conference. She pointed out to us that her patients come from the urban terraces of cities in the north-west of England and have never had 'sensory gardens'. They are much more likely to have had a backyard with a washing line and perhaps a pigeon loft. She and Kate Andrews used triggers to stimulate discussion amongst people with dementia about their memories of nature; and many of the memories were about growing food in hard times during the war. Many of her respondents talked about parks; others mentioned other places such as:

> 'Used to go up near the railway line as there were swans there.'

Or:

> 'Used to take the bairns down to the cemetery for a walk.'

They make several suggestions, one of which is that the outside spaces of care homes for these life-long urban dwellers might usefully look more like a park.

Nature for reminiscence

James McKillop's memories of his childhood contacts with nature demonstrate how vivid they are. James is 72 and has dementia, but he can lucidly describe exploring nature in the local wood once he was big and strong enough to get over the dyke, and his sense of wonder at things such as the luminescent skin of the newts. James is an accomplished photographer and many of his photographs are of natural things such as dandelion clocks; clearly a feature of his childhood. There must be hundreds of men with dementia with these vivid memories that are seldom stirred by the usual reminiscence materials.

Person-centred care is culturally sensitive care

As we said earlier, we asked Joan Domicelj to contribute because of her knowledge of numerous ancient cultures and the landscapes that are important to them, particularly the aboriginal people of Australia.

She makes some very important observations about the universal and the familiar and about the experience of being a migrant:

> The familiar offers comfort; displacement from usual surroundings is a challenge. The presence of earth, sky and life around us may be constant but their fluctuating characteristics are not. Migrants experience disorientation when moved out of their normal surroundings; people with dementia even more poignantly.

If we think about cultures so very different from our own, we are better alerted to the need to think about all differences and the need to tailor care to the individual. We need to understand that it is often the belief systems and interpretations that are different – even of the same aspects of nature. Beth Britton's father, for example, had a deeply physical relationship with the land. Nature is important to look at but also to experience physically and with our senses.

We are really most grateful to all our contributors for providing us with such thoughtful contributions.

Final thoughts

Nature remains important for everyone, however disabled by dementia, and not just for its health benefits. Being outside both enables us to lose our identities, which can be very therapeutic for people who resent being 'a person who is cared for', and sometimes to enjoy another identity such as being good at growing vegetables. Nature is also non-judgemental. Everyone enjoys it in their own way without criticism or any sense of success or failure. This must be very helpful to people who feel very lacking in confidence.

As editors, we are aware that our interest in nature and dementia is only in part a reaction to research that shows how deprived of it many people with dementia are. It is also in part because the whole world is waking up to the importance of seeing humans as part of nature with a responsibility for looking after it in a way that benefits the whole.

Richard Louv (2011) calls this the Nature Principle: 'The future will belong to the nature-smart – those individuals, families, businesses, and political leaders who develop a deeper understanding of the transformative power of the natural world and who balance the virtual with the real. The more high-tech we become, the more nature we need.'

The aim of this book is to get people with dementia outside in contact with nature more often, by making outside areas and outside experiences more familiar to them. In this way we can re-awaken those intense, elemental, simple and vivid memories of nature in childhood. We want to forge a link which is often broken between people with dementia and nature. We believe this is possible even when people are unable to go outside because they are too sick, because nature can be brought in to them in various ways. We believe that if we have a deeper understanding of cultural differences in the widest sense we can reconnect people with dementia to something very deep and important in all of us. We hope this book is a contribution to making this happen.

A Family's Perspective on Nature and Dementia

Using the Great Outdoors to Help the Inner Person

BETH BRITTON

My father loved being outside. In fact I would say it was where he was at his happiest and most relaxed, which is no great surprise since in his working life he had been a farmer and, when he was not tending his cattle, a keen gardener. Dad was a traditionalist, everything you would imagine an Englishman born into a Norfolk farming family would be. During his working life even his appearance exuded his upbringing as he walked the fields in his trademark collared shirt, braces, tweed cap and with baler twine keeping his trousers firmly placed inside his wellington boots.

Dad's love of animals and the countryside was a huge feature of my childhood. One of my earliest memories of spending time with Dad is the vivid recollection of me bottle feeding two lambs he had brought home one day, their enthusiasm for the milk almost knocking me over. Or the time when he had a mole in the palm of his hand and carefully showed it to me, explaining about how it used its feet to dig holes and make mole hills.

During my childhood I would spend many hours waiting patiently in the car on the farm when Dad had veterinary work to do with his cattle that made it unsafe for me to be in the yard, whilst on other days I would be helping him carry bags of feed across the fields. Family mealtimes around the dining table would often feature Dad talking about animals that he had cared for, prizes he had won and how modern agriculture was so different to the experiences of his youth.

My father was a huge advocate of sustainable farming, preserving nature and working in harmony with the land. He had numerous books on the subject and throughout his working life he always tried to practise what he preached. When he was not with his animals he would be found on his allotment, growing enough vegetables and fruits for his family to last us all year round. Produced organically, not only were they delicious and a feature of every meal from the moment I was given solid food, to my young and enquiring mind they represented something amazing. How a small seed could produce something I could eat seemed miraculous, so Dad set about feeding my enthusiasm with knowledge and first-hand experience until I was pestering him for my own corner of the garden to grow plants.

Every one of those passions and beliefs never left Dad when he developed vascular dementia; indeed, I would say that memories of his earlier life became even stronger and more important. What did change, however, was his ability to interact with his passions. He had dementia for about 19 years, for the first ten of which he went without a diagnosis, and it was during that decade that his struggles to look after himself and his home began to impact upon the things that he loved the most.

His garden became overgrown, to the point where it was almost like a jungle. The fruits went unpicked, the vegetable seeds were never sown. More worryingly, because he had always grown his own fruit and veg rather than buying them, he had no concept of the need to purchase what he was no longer producing and so his diet suffered. He would sit indoors, with the windows closed and the curtains drawn, surrounded by the books he loved but no longer read, with a head full of memories mixed with vivid imaginations of what he thought was happening around him.

For a man who so loved being outside, this was uncharacteristic to say the least. In hindsight, although it was partly due to the problems he was having with his joints that made long periods of standing up impossible, it was far more attributable to what we now know was his dementia. He lost the ability to not only understand what he needed to do, but to have the concentration to do it. In the end he tried to block it out by keeping the curtains shut to stop himself being reminded, and his pride prevented him from allowing us to help.

When Dad's health suddenly deteriorated and he had to move into care, the task of sorting out his possessions brought an unexpected gem to life. For many years during my childhood Dad had been jotting down his thoughts on farming and the countryside. He had written copious notes about the experiences from his youth and descriptions of East Anglian landscapes, but unbeknown to me he had also been recording them. One such recording is Dad talking at length about when he got his call-up papers. He described how his first reaction was to flee down through the fields to a stream to be at one with nature, do some fishing and contemplate how being in the army would compare with his life of rural contentment.

Given that we discovered this recording at a time when Dad was unable to hold a coherent conversation with us, listening to him talking so lucidly, passionately and with such intricate descriptions of insects and scenery was fascinating. It was the landscape and lifestyle of his youth, and it represented an era that his dementia had now taken him back to. It served as a very timely reminder that whilst his carers were concerned about keeping him securely inside a building and meeting his needs within those walls, a huge part of Dad's actual need was to remain in touch with the natural elements in modern life that could still connect him to his younger days.

My father would go on to spend the last nine years of his life in care homes, punctuated by spells in hospital, all of which were many miles away from his Norfolk roots. Early on in his journey through the care system, when Dad was still walking and talking and getting himself into all kinds of scrapes, he would tell the care staff about needing to milk his cattle, and other tales of day-to-day life as a farmer. From his early months in care homes, through to just a few weeks before he passed away, Dad wanted to be outside. Never once when he was asked did he refuse to go, and indeed while he was mobile he often attempted to open the locked doors himself.

We deliberately chose a room on the ground floor of the care home, specifically because we wanted Dad to remain connected with the outdoor life that he had always loved. It was to prove imperative, however, that we as a family facilitated the simple act of him being allowed outside. Indoors my father was imprisoned; largely for his own good admittedly (after all, no one wanted him getting lost and ending up on the road), but this led to him becoming very frustrated. In hot and stuffy conditions, where stale food smells lingered, escaping other residents for some time alone was almost impossible and conflicting electronic sounds filled the air, my father must have felt like he was being tortured.

For a man used to hearing birdsong and insects buzzing, cattle mooing, lambs bleating and cockerels waking the neighbourhood, it was a cultural change that only served to make his dementia symptoms more pronounced. He could not orientate himself in such an unfamiliar environment, and given that he was someone who valued independence and generally preferred the company of farmyard animals to humans, it was like putting him on a ride at a crowded fair and never letting him off.

Whilst it may appear easier to run a care home where all the residents are sat around the edge of a room, a TV is put on and minimal supervision is required from staff members, what actually happens is that all perceptions of time of day and time of year become lost for those people. They never feel the changing temperatures or the differences in the weather, and they never get to appreciate the landscape in all of its seasonal glories.

Enabling people to breathe fresh air, to hear the rustling trees and the tweeting birds, to hold and smell the flowers and to feel the wind in their hair and the sun on their face requires thoughtful planning, and often more staffing. You also need outdoor spaces that are accessible for residents with different mobility needs, displaying various behaviours, having particular likes and dislikes, and with numerous expectations of what they would want from going outside.

For example, my father went from walking independently to going everywhere by wheelchair, so the garden became inaccessible to him for a while until it had been landscaped with suitable pathways. When he could still walk he was in danger of trying to go beyond the parameter of the garden and into the neighbouring fields, particularly when the horses were out and he wanted to be closer to them. In his wheelchair, he was completely dependent on others to facilitate him going outside and then being taken closer to the things that would interest him.

Without a family, my father would have been lucky to go outside possibly once a month during the summer. Despite making the garden suitable for the differing needs of the residents, with pathways around the largest area and a smaller contained section nearest to the building that could help to keep residents who liked to walk secure whilst still being able to enjoy the raised beds and tubs of plants, the garden went largely unused.

Going outside was not a formal part of the activities programme – the yearly garden party or fête would often be held indoors, and at one time staff were even forbidden from taking their lunch breaks outside. Residents, when they were brought from their rooms to the lounge, would usually be sat around the television with the French doors to the garden closed. At mealtimes, as the TV still blared out, the curtains would often be shut too.

Our approach as a family, however, was very different and far more proactive. When Dad could no longer walk we would phone ahead of our visit to request that he be helped into a wheelchair ready to go outside. If it was a mealtime, we would make it clear that we would also be helping him to eat his food outside. On our arrival Dad would be ready for his adventure, and whilst over time his dementia robbed him of the ability to articulate his relief at being reunited with nature, his body language said it all.

Suddenly Dad would be more alert; he would follow the movement of the plants or turn his head for the song a bird was singing. Even sounds not associated with the natural world, such as cars going past or planes overhead, captured his attention. Sometimes sights or sounds would surprise him, possibly even startle him. Yet even in the moments where his thoughts were interrupted or his snoozing was disturbed, his reaction was of a man happy to have experienced the unexpected.

Going outside instantly changed his day, from something predictable and boring to something where every movement or sound represented life outside of the incarceration he experienced indoors. Looking at the same four walls hour after hour, unable to articulate himself as he once had, with his mind taking on a different identity as he gradually lost control over his life, must have been hell for my father. Putting him back in touch with something as timeless as the outside world was like a reconnection with the man he was, the man he still remembered being.

Sadly he was often alone in this experience, with other residents only occasionally joining us despite their love of outdoor spaces being well known. There was another man who had been a farmer and always revelled in his very brief and occasional forays outside, whilst the family of a female resident openly admitted that she had loved the outdoors her whole life. They reminisced about how she used to sit out in all weathers, and that she would have felt like a 'caged bird' as a result of being kept inside.

Sometimes residents who liked to walk would be brought down from upstairs to pace the garden with a carer, but those opportunities were few and far between. Thus our experience of Dad's years in a care homes was that whilst we would sit outside with him enjoying sunshine and fresh air, other residents, even those with visiting families, would be kept inside and not even offered the chance to go into the garden or further afield.

All of this begs an important question – when do people living in a care home have the sensation of their heart beating a little faster in harmony with the outside world? Unless you actually expose them to something the rest of us take for granted they will never have that. It is an isolated, unrealistic and very sad way to live. Moreover, by failing to appreciate the need to remain connected with the world around them, those caring for people with dementia are contributing to the mental decline associated with this disease.

Of course, there is so much more to utilising outdoor spaces than just sitting and observing. Whilst passive enjoyment is very important, bringing with it relaxation and contentment, gardens are also interactive places where people with dementia can be encouraged and facilitated to participate in growing and tending plants. At my father's care home raised beds were built into the garden, but residents were never given the opportunity to grow their own fruits and vegetables, something that would have brought back such precious memories for my father. Initially there was a small kitchen garden, but it was something that staff and volunteers created and maintained for a short period of time before the attempts to grow edible plants were abandoned in favour of seasonal flowers.

For my father the great outdoors was also the obvious venue for social occasions. Not only would we have family meals outside and tea parties together, but birthdays were also celebrated and we even had an Easter egg hunt. Eating outside has huge advantages for people with dementia, not least because fresh air is very stimulating for what can often be flagging appetites amongst the older generation.

We did not just confine this activity to the care home grounds either. Since in Dad's case it was impossible for the care home to provide every form of outdoor stimulation that he needed (sadly we could not have a farmyard in the garden!), we took him on trips out of the home. Not only did this provide the chance to experience different views and sensations on the journey, but in the case of the farm we visited, he would arrive in a place that had animals he instantly recognised. Touching them, hearing their familiar cries and smelling the farmyard environment was far more natural to my father than anything he experienced within the walls of his care home.

The same was true of our last visit with Dad to a local woodland. The rustling trees, the crisp autumn leaves crushing under the weight of his wheelchair and the fresh clean smell in the air as we kept our gloved hands warm around mugs of hot tea all resulted in the biggest smile on Dad's face, and body language that betrayed sheer unadulterated contentment. Harvest and autumn time was always a favourite with my father, and by wrapping up warmly he was able to go out and experience a season that offers such unique sounds and aromas.

I would be the first to admit that we never truly succeeded in re-creating Dad's childhood memories of East Anglian landscapes that were well beyond a distance that he could reasonably travel. However, we ensured that elements from that time were present all around him throughout his journey with dementia. Often it was the smallest details, things that perhaps would never normally register with us in our busy lives, that brought the strongest reaction from Dad. They became inspirational in our quest to bring his memories alive. Indeed, it was only during the times when he was in hospital that he was totally denied access to this type of stimulation, and the effect on him was a very negative one.

Sharing outdoor experiences with Dad, knowing how much they meant to him, was a very enriching experience for us as his family.

On the many occasions we were sat outside with my father, those times also provided a valuable insight for his carers into what made him truly happy and contented. The continually changing outdoor environment stimulated conversation, and enabled us to talk to Dad about things that we knew he loved, like roses for example, whilst actually holding, feeling and smelling them.

Within a building the dementia care environment can be a very stressful one, not only for the person with dementia but also for those who are caring for them or visiting them. When you move the experience of caring for someone outside, it reduces those stress levels immeasurably. It also promotes learning, and puts you into a continually changing natural landscape that everyone shares on the same level.

Although in so many ways my father's dementia represented a huge daily struggle for him, it also protected him from the passage of change that, even when I was a child, he highlighted negatively in farming practices and the use of chemicals. The last place my father farmed is now a new housing development. It would have broken his heart to watch the construction of those properties on land that was once fertile pasture, with winding streams, water meadows, hedgerows, insects and wild flowers.

That type of natural environment was always my father's real home. It was a place where his human spirit connected with the universe in a way that was timeless. It was something he would have strived to protect and defend before his dementia developed, and something that he needed to be kept in touch with during his time in care. In a communal setting there are so many different interpretations of what makes an outdoor space something that is reminiscent of the residents' former lives – from people who grew up playing on perfectly manicured lawns surrounded by topiary, to people like my father, who embraced the natural world and all its irregularities.

Looking beyond the residents you have in a care home at any one time, and into the future where you may have people with very different memories, means that many homes design their outdoor spaces to be generally acceptable for everyone, with tactile plants, fragrant flowers, water features and winding pathways. Yet even in these functional spaces, finding the elements that make it relevant to the person you are caring for can be an exciting and challenging voyage of discovery.

Just as being in a garden frees a person from the confines of a building, so gardens have their boundaries. In terms of outdoor experiences, true personalisation for my father was only found by looking further afield and planning trips away from the care home. We found a world on our doorstep that provided very enriching experiences for Dad and, combined with the time he spent in the garden at the care home, contributed to the happiest and most memorable occasions we had with him.

Naturally, when Dad passed away in April 2012 there was only one setting that could be his final resting place – a beautiful churchyard bordering a stable yard, overlooking rolling hills and countryside, with villages dotted in the distance, horses grazing in the fields and rabbits running amuck. It represents everything he truly loved: his happiest days, his strongest memories and the most perfect example of a little corner of England that will be forever his.

Chapter 2

Nature for People with Dementia in Japan

Some Examples of Horticultural Activities in Japanese Care Homes

YUTAKA INOUE

Japanese seasons

Japanese people are considered as nature loving, due particularly to the fact that the four seasons are very distinct from each other in Japan. The spring begins with 'ume' or Japanese apricot flowers, which are the themes of many Japanese paintings as well as Japanese short poems. After ume comes the season of 'sakura' or cherry blossoms, under which many people gather to have picnics with food and drink which sometimes makes them jolly. In Japan, the weather forecast usually involves the forecast for the time of various degrees of bloom of the sakura in various regions.

The end of spring is marked by days of long drizzling rains with occasional sunny days which ultimately bring about the very hot and often sultry Japanese summer. In recent years, the summers have become hotter and hotter due to global warming. People become lethargic in the hot days. But many grand festivals in various parts in Japan take place in summer.

The summer ends also with a rainy season as well as occasional typhoons. The autumn is considered by many as the best season with a temperate atmosphere and blue skies often without a single cloud. In the old days, people gathered and admired the dramatic rise of the full moon, which was conspicuous in this clear weather. The autumn is the season when leaves change their colors. Even today, excursions are very popular for viewing 'momiji' or Japanese scarlet maples which aflame the hills and valleys.

The Japanese winter is quite different according to the region, due to the seasonal chilly winds which come from Siberia over the Sea of Japan. They bring consecutive days of heavy snow to the north-western side of the central ridges in Japan, while leaving the Pacific side, including metropolitan areas, almost always very sunny and dry with little snow or rain.

Japanese dwellings

When Japanese people talk about nature, they are often talking about the seasonal features they see around their dwellings. As shown in the life of plants and flowers, cicadas and butterflies, or migratory birds, in the minds of most Japanese people, including people with dementia, nature and the seasons are supposed to be intertwined. It should be added that many modern high-rise apartment buildings made of reinforced concrete sometimes have large sliding glass doors and windows which are wide open to balconies, reflecting this Japanese tradition.

Traditional Japanese houses are made of timber with a number of sliding doors which can be wide open during the hot summer to allow ventilation. There exist almost no masonry structures, due less to the climate than to the frequent earthquakes. So, traditional Japanese houses are not air-tight at all, with inevitable cold drafts in the winter.

Care homes of the hospital or institutional building type, however, are an environment which is quite different from family dwellings, apart from group homes which in Japan are normally very homelike but often lack necessary design features for frail elderly people using wheelchairs.

In what follows, I would like to present some care home settings, including group homes for people with dementia, which practice horticultural therapy as a major part of their therapeutic (or preventative) activities. (I use the word 'preventative' because, in Japan, activities are thought to have preventative qualities in terms of the progress of dementia.)

Diversionary therapy introduced from Australia

Yukarigaoka is in a commuting residential area on the outskirts of Tokyo which has been developed since the 1980s. As its residents are getting older, the developer has built various types of care home for frail older residents, including people with dementia. They have been built around a fairly large garden at the fringe of the development. At the moment, there are three types of care home: 'tokuyo' (nursing homes provided by the social sector[1]), 'roken' (intermediate nursing homes for rehabilitation), and group homes (group living for people with dementia). There are also some apartment-type dwellings with care services being built for independent older people. They are located in the central area near the train station and shopping facilities.

I would like to explain the therapeutic activities provided in the roken and the group home. As discussed later, it appears that there are few outdoor activities taking place in tokuyos. As the name of the area 'Eucalypti Hills' indicates, the developer has had contacts with Australia and has introduced therapeutic activities widely practiced in Australia. Mr. Yamaguchi, who is responsible for the therapeutic activities at the roken as well as the management and maintenance of the garden, had undertaken training in diversionary therapy in Brisbane. He said that he found some cultural differences between Australia and Japan with respect to old people's attitude towards nature: 'In Australia, residents seemed interested in tending plants and flowers, whereas in Japan, many residents look happy just to observe the seasonal changes in nature and to be moving around in the garden.'

The aim of the roken is to rehabilitate the residents so they become independent and able to live in their homes again. So, they have prepared and scheduled many indoor and outdoor activities for rehabilitation as well as to interest the residents. There are many outdoor activities taking place in the garden: tending flowers, planting various vegetables, cropping bamboo shoots, and even keeping bees. Once a month, domestic animals – for example, ponies and rabbits –

---

[1]   Tokuyos are allowed to be established and run by local authorities and authorized non-profit organizations only. The buildings and staff arrangements are strictly controlled and their construction and running costs are heavily subsidized.

are brought from an animal farm to the garden. On the day when I visited, Mr. Yamaguchi was preparing equipment for mini-golf with large wooden balls, wood putters and big holes which was planned to take place in the field in the afternoon. Although residents are expected to stay in rokens for a relatively short period, it appears that most residents were staying as long as two or three years, due mainly to the shortage in the number of tokuyos (nursing homes). Seventy per cent of this roken's residents had some degree of dementia.

There is a bungalow care home facing the garden specifically for group living for people with dementia. This building has two units, each housing nine residents. In the center at the entrance there is a fairly large nursery room for the schoolchildren living in this area.[2] So, the group home residents can have contact with another kind of nature: 30–40 children playing. Mr. Suzuki, the manager of the group home, said that even naughty children were sometimes very kind to the old people, accepting the people with dementia as they are. They sometimes helped staff to locate the residents, as the residents were free to go outside and the children were playing at the entrance. Although children and old people do not normally talk to each other very much or play together, they seem to have good relationships. The residents of the group home can go out to the large garden with various trees, bamboos, and flowers, and also beyond the garden to neighborhood areas at any time, because the garden is open to the public.

They are also invited to participate in the activities prepared by the roken, such as harvesting vegetables and contact with animals. It appears that the residents have not shown any significant therapeutic benefit from the contacts with animals, but they seemed happy with the diversionary activities, especially the people who used to work in gardens or farms. They seem to enjoy especially cooking the vegetables they have picked.

---

2   In Japan there is a statutory system of Gakudo Hoiku (literally translated as schoolchild nursing) for school boys and girls whose parents or relatives are absent from home after school. Special staff are assigned to provide activities including tea time with sweets.

A small group home practicing horticultural activities

'Kaju' is a small building which looks similar to the dwellings nearby in the residential area near Kamakura, the ancient capital of Japan. Eighteen residents with dementia live here. The building is designed for a group of nine people on the ground floor and nine on the upper floor. It is not specially designed for frail elderly people apart from some handrails in the halls, corridors, bathrooms, and some other places. Sitting areas are small and rather cramped, as are the bedrooms, which are not only small but have no en-suite facilities. Communal bathrooms are too small for residents using wheelchairs or requiring extensive care and help, let alone terminal care. So, the residents, once they become too ill or frail and are needing continuous medical treatment and care, are supposed to be moved to other nursing homes or hospitals. Few residents live there longer than five years. However, the oldest resident was 99 years old when I visited.

There are two gardens where therapeutic activities take place. They are not very much larger than those of many Japanese detached houses. In the front garden there are raised flower beds, many flower planters, and two benches. In the rather narrow back garden they grow various vegetables, although there are no special staff for gardening activities apart from the manager of the home, Mr. Katsumata. Many students and some teachers from a nearby gardening school are involved, since the school is run by the owner of this home. At times, they guide residents to walk to the nearby park or to some other places with big trees. It appears that some neighborhood schoolchildren and volunteers are also involved in these activities and seasonal events.

Mr. Katsumata said that residents are very fond of being outdoors and engaging in gardening activities, but they were unreliable in tending plants and flowers due to memory impairment. The residents used to go out into the gardens whenever they liked, as in many Japanese group homes, but after recurring incidents in which they had to ask the police to find lost residents the front door of this group home has been locked.

A luxury retirement community practicing horticultural activities

'Comfort Azamino' is a complex three-storey building of barrier-free apartments and two nursing home units in the suburbs of Tokyo, about 20 minutes by train from the metropolitan central area. Because of its location as well as the standard of the building with various gardens around it and carefully worked-out care services, it is considered as one of the best as well as the most expensive retirement homes in Japan for rich elderly people who want to live their remaining years in comfort and without any worries about care. Once residents become too frail to stay independently in their apartment, they can move to the nursing home attached to this complex building with 24-hour constant care.

In the land-scarce country of Japan, and especially in a heavily populated metropolitan area, the most salient feature of this complex building lies in the seven gardens placed between and around the wings. Each garden has its own character and is named, such as 'village garden', with such nostalgic Japanese landscape features as a rice paddy field and a water mill, or 'sunset garden', planted with white flowers which are supposed to be more beautiful at sunset and at dusk. These gardens were designed by a famous professor of landscape architecture, who made the best use of native vegetation as well as quite extensive planting. Varieties are so many that even the horticultural therapist that I interviewed, Mr. Matsui, could not list all of them. Some flowers are such rare native species that you cannot find them even in large florists in Tokyo. There are flowers all year round, though fewer flowers are seen in winter, mainly Christmas roses. Since the opening of this building in 2006, Mr. Matsui has tried to train volunteers to take care of the plants in the gardens, and there are now 17 volunteers.

Various horticultural therapeutic activities, such as planting and harvesting of rice, making pressed flowers, or arranging floral decorations for Christmas, are organized by Mr. Matsui twice a month for a group of residents. Residents are encouraged to bring plants from their previous homes, especially when they feel some special attachment to them. They are planted in the garden or placed on the balconies where they can look at them from their apartments. Some residents bring back the plants used in the therapeutic activities to their apartment balconies.

In addition to the group activities, Mr. Matsui undertakes individually tailored therapies in the garden with the help of the care staff. He says that one of the good things about involving care staff in the gardens is that not only residents but also the staff seem to become happier due to the improved relationships nurtured by the gardening activities. Although it is difficult to ascertain any effects of the horticultural therapies quantitatively, he has gained the definite impression that just to look at plants which very slowly change their shapes and colors can bring about stability in residents' minds, and more positive attitudes.

Of the precise records of various activities for each resident which Mr. Matsui keeps, I would like to present the following three cases as examples of what has happened to the residents with respect to the horticultural therapies or activities in the gardens.

The first case is Mr. A., who lost his wife two years after moving into this retirement community. He was so depressed that he totally confined himself indoors. He had lost his circadian rhythm to such a degree that he often appeared in the dining room in the evenings to have breakfast. However, since he used to love horticultural activities when he and his wife were at their previous home, he took part in the therapeutic activities, such as planting flowers, picking vegetables, and making New Year decorations, with the result that he resumed his former daily rhythm and got over the mourning period for the death of his wife.

The second case is Ms. B., who has dementia. She used to be a very active person and had worked for a long time to help women by establishing and running nurseries. After she got dementia, it was discovered that she used to write haiku. Haiku is a Japanese short poem consisting of only 17 syllables. Although she has been steadily losing her memory, she is leading an active life by making haiku once again. In every haiku there must be a 'kigo', a predetermined word with which a seasonal feature is associated. One often finds nature in haiku, for example plants and animals associated with the season. So, one day a member of staff took her out for a walk in the gardens. Since then she often goes out to look at flowers and trees to make haiku. Sometimes she takes pictures of them. At party events held in the community, she often presents her haiku and pictures. As a result, many residents and staff now regard her with respect as an artist.

Examples of tanka (verses with 31 syllables) and haiku (verses with 17 syllables) written by Ms. B. and translated by me are:

> As silent night deepens,
> I watched all on my own
> a hazy moon,
> with remembrances
> of my old days.

> Looking up at sky
> without a cloud,
> I longed for
> my old home on the coast
> with a view of azure ocean.

> Cherishing the summer
> passing away…
> singings of crickets
> autumn is deepening:
> I see red dragonflies
> high in the sky.

The third case is Ms. C., who has always been grumbling and complaining about the services she receives in this community, due in part to the high expectations she has for the high fees she pays, as well as some other causes. The staff had been very worried and embarrassed about her but did not know how to deal with this situation. One day she received a bougainvillea as a present from her son who she had not got along with very well. However, she reared and tended the flower with the utmost care and then started therapeutic gardening activities. Since then, she seems to have gained peace of mind with much less grumbling.

Conclusion and discussion

Although Japan is prone to natural disasters, as evidenced by the recent earthquakes and subsequent tsunamis as well as occasional typhoons, the people of Japan and nature are in close contact. This is due not only to the temperate climate with distinctive seasonal features, but also to the traditional design of Japanese dwellings which are wide open to nature.

For people with dementia to have sufficient contact with nature in today's care home environment, however, there should be adequate accessible outdoor spaces and staffing to assist contact. The outdoor spaces should be designed and maintained as enjoyable gardens, which require skills and labor. To assist the residents to enjoy the outdoor activities, skills and work are needed too, either by staff or volunteers.

So far have presented three types of care home environment for people with dementia in which therapeutic activities are practiced in the gardens:

- one intermediate nursing home for rehabilitation (roken)
- two group homes for people with dementia
- one retirement community.

In Yukarigaoka, a roken and a group home, which are run by the same owner, not only have a large common garden but also employ specialist staff for the therapeutic activities. 'Kaju', a group home, has only small gardens but is run in association with a gardening school. 'Comfort Azamino', a retirement community, has various gardens and special staff for the horticultural therapy. All these environments involve a number of volunteers for the gardening activities. In these environments, contact with nature from gardening activities seems to bring about enhanced happiness and peace of mind to the residents, although these effects are not quite measurable.

Compared with these environments, tokuyos, the most common type of nursing care home in Japan provided by the social sector for frail elderly people, including people with dementia, are typically places where residents are confined inside and can seldom go outside, even if there are outdoor spaces including balconies or roof gardens. Designs of most tokuyos use hospital or institutional building models lacking homelike features or decor. Their staff are always busy assisting residents with their daily lives, including bathing in the bath tubs and drinking water after the bath, as Japanese elderly people very often prefer a long and hot bath.

As the Japanese population is rapidly aging, there are long waiting times for tokuyos in many areas, especially densely populated metropolitan regions. There do exist some tokuyos providing more person-centered care and maintaining good relationships with their neighborhood, including recruiting volunteers for activities or events. However, assisting residents to go outside is beyond their resources, due in part to the buildings themselves which are normally too big, and they have not given due consideration on how to prepare and use outdoor spaces.

Chapter 3

Getting Out and About in the British Countryside

Dementia Adventure

NEIL MAPES

Introduction

I was about six years old when dementia entered our family life. Our family has deep roots within rural farming communities near Chelmsford in Essex, stretching back for at least the last two hundred years. In a book about cultural differences I share the story of my grandparents here to add to the colour and breadth of experiences and as an introduction to why Dementia Adventure began. I recall dancing purples and leaping greens which made up the mesmerising natural display in my grandparents' fireplace. I also remember sitting far too close, the burning willow spitting like a firecracker, adding to the fun of the fire. But perhaps most vivid of all in my memory is the smell of the wood fire. A log fire glowing in the hearth is both elemental and central to many people's childhood memories. For many the hearth is the centre of the experience we call home. Most of the world still cooks on wood fires, but in Britain most people have lost a connection with nature in that they have 'forgotten' how to lay a wood fire.

I remember my grandparents Vic and Annie as strong country people. Annie made jam after spells gathering fruit from the hedgerows and Vic would spend hours gardening and collecting wood on local farmland for burning on the fire. I remember sitting around the fire with Annie and Vic, with Vic shouting at Giant Haystacks wrestling on the telly and Annie laughing – happy family memories. Annie and Vic both subsequently lived with and died with dementia. Annie was starting to show signs of dementia when I was about six years old. Vic's dementia symptoms showed first when I was about 13. Right up until his death he was collecting and chopping up firewood from the fields, to such an extent that he had literally 'shed-loads' of firewood.

I now have a six-year-old son and a two-year-old daughter, and perhaps unsurprisingly I have a wood fire, which our family sit around in the autumn and winter, repeating the delightful and generational fireside memory. Instead of an open fire we have a wood-burning stove. The wood-burning stove is seemingly a very middle-class fascination, and its popularity in recent times I believe is indicative of a fundamental unhappiness I see in a lot of Britain today. We own more things and have more stuff, certainly more technology, and yet life seems ever more complex and we appear to lack 'quality time'. I believe there are a growing number of people searching for a simpler life, one which reminds us of our deep cultural memories, of the romantic rural idyll, of 'life in the good old days'. We cannot of course go back to those days, nor were some of them good, mainly because our population is growing and ageing, and more people like Annie and Vic are getting dementia.

Dementia Adventure was set up after supporting Annie and Vic and my mum and subsequently hundreds of other families living with dementia stretching over a 15-year period. Fundamentally we want to offer people more choices and more opportunities to get out into nature. We started with a simple mission: to connect people living with dementia to nature and a sense of adventure. The complexities of the range of dementias are still becoming fully understood, and whilst we wait for medical advances to bring us news of a cure, connecting with nature is arguably one of the most easily accessible evidence-based therapies (for more information on the evidence base please visit www.greenexercise.org or the Dementia Adventure website research pages, given at the end of this chapter), enabling people with dementia to have a 'life worth living'. We will share here some of our nature-based adventures which took place in 2012 and highlight how we can maintain our personal and emotional connection with nature, despite having dementia.

Nature-based adventures

Our adventure provision takes a variety of forms, but is centrally concerned with supporting people to share and enjoy activity together out in nature. Our work at Dementia Adventure has three levels. Ideally we aim to get people active out in nature. If we cannot do that, simply getting people out of buildings into nature (even if only for five minutes) is good enough. And the third level of our work is to bring nature into buildings, into the lives of people who spend all of their day indoors. A hearth or wood-burning stove is one way of doing this, as are real plants that people can look after and nurture. Bringing nature inside is perhaps a topic to explore more fully another time; we will concentrate here on our first level of work: activity outdoors.

We designed and led a variety of nature-based adventures in 2012. We will share and reflect on how these activities say something important about our British cultural identity. The adventures themselves include:

1. park walks

2. woodland celebration days

3. hands-on sailing holidays.

All our provision is carefully designed and thoroughly researched. We carry out risk–benefit assessments on all of our adventures and directly support the adventures with our own staff and volunteers. People living with dementia and their family carers often generate the original idea for the adventures and are consulted on how to design and deliver the adventure as well as reviewing its impact and success. We have specialist insurance cover, support people to access specialist personal travel insurance, and have developed a successful model of adventure provision. This model ensures that there are more people on the adventure without dementia than there are with dementia – safety in numbers. The model also includes issuing a special invitation and motivation to get out into nature, a personalised experience with choices on the adventure and creating a 'dementia-friendly' environment.

So far, younger people and people in the earlier stages of dementia have been attracted by our sailing holidays and activity breaks. A typical holiday will involve 12 people: four people living with dementia, four family carers and four staff and/or volunteers. People who are further down the road in their dementia journey, many of whom are living in care homes, have so far benefited from our park walks and woodland days out. However, some care home providers recently have expressed interest in some of their residents being supported to go on holiday – a very positive development.

Park walks

Parks and publicly accessible green open spaces are often close to home, even in urban centres. If we aren't walking the dog then we are there with our children or running around the park as part of a charitable fundraising event. Britain also has a long and diverse history in designing, managing and opening up access to parks and public green spaces for us all to enjoy. It is perhaps the first and easiest step to physically getting ourselves out into nature. For the British middle classes there has been a trend towards supporting the award-winning gardens and parkland through membership to highly managed and cultivated green spaces. Yet for decades we have delighted in sitting on the green lawns (when allowed) and smelling the roses in many parks and taking tips (and cuttings) from the horticultural elite which we can put into place in our own gardens.

Dementia Adventure has delivered supported park walks for people living with dementia for the last three years. Participants include people living in their own homes, who often simply want to walk as much as they can, as well as people living with more advanced stages of dementia in care homes. People come on walks with Dementia Adventure because they are near to home and are designed with people living with dementia in mind and are supported walks. Everyone is in the same boat and there is safety in numbers attending a led walk.

In Essex we recently led a weekly programme of ten park walks in the summer months which were attended by 208 people who enjoyed 312 hours out in nature (each walk being 90 minutes long). Below are some quotes from participants in those walks and walks we have led elsewhere in England.

From people living with dementia

'I like to walk as much is allowed.'

'I had a good day.'

'I had the best ice cream.'

'This is the best day.'

'Walks are a lot of fun.'

From care home staff

'These walks have enhanced the lives of our residents immensely, enabling them to experience being in a different environment, and also to socialise with others who suffer from the various stages of dementia. It was also good for our staff members to chat with care staff from other homes, to gain ideas and also learn of their experiences. It has been so rewarding for care staff and family to see the pleasure it has given our residents.'

'We don't usually get much response from the resident but he seemed to come alive on this visit.'

'One resident said he had an overwhelming feeling of camaraderie, a sense of belonging.'

'A resident was able to identify trees and flowers. I didn't know what they were.'

'It was nice for the residents to be with so many people.'

'Family carers were able to enjoy the visit without the stress of having to look after their loved one.'

From family carers

'You could see the residents were enjoying it.'

'It was Mum as I always knew her; I had her back with me again.'

'I'd like to do more visits of this kind.'

Woodland celebration days

Hundreds of years ago all Britain would have been ancient woodland. Ancestrally we have come from the woods, but today Britain's woods are in decline and are often neglected and under threat from various 'development' plans. Yet amazingly, according to the Woodland Trust, over half of the people in Britain still live within 4km of a wood (www.visitwoods.org.uk). We recently delivered a training day for green space organisations in Epping Forest, which is a great example of the type of woodland which would have once covered our islands. We owe it to ourselves, to our heritage and to our future generations to celebrate the gifts of woodland. The Woodland Trust is a charity which aims to protect native trees and woods, as well as planting more trees and inspiring people to visit woods. Dementia Adventure has worked with the VisitWoods team at the Woodland Trust on a succession of projects. One of these in 2012 was our woodland celebration day.

On 24 July 2012 Dementia Adventure convened 77 people, including 38 people living with dementia, who enjoyed a day of activity out in nature at Lochore Meadows in Scotland. The day was also blessed by sunshine. Participants came from a variety of backgrounds and included family members and carers from residential and nursing homes as well as active younger groups of people living with dementia. A variety of nature activities were on offer for people with different interests and with varying levels of need and frailty. People living with dementia using wheelchairs enjoyed the picnic lunch, views across the lake, nature noughts and crosses, recording their connection with nature on strips of cotton (see below), as well as reminiscing about the location and elements of nature from their younger days. Some of the participants remembered the coal mine which stood on the site before the planting of the woodland, whilst others reminisced about family days out enjoyed as children. Indoor activities were also on offer for people to make nature collages. The more physically able participants enjoyed these activities as well as a loch-side walk, with a small group taking an extended walk around the woodland.

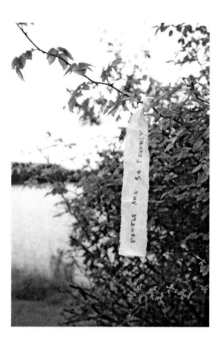

Figure 3.1 Woodland Celebration with the Woodland Trust Scotland

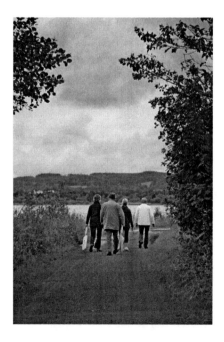

Figure 3.2 Woodland Celebration with the Woodland Trust Scotland

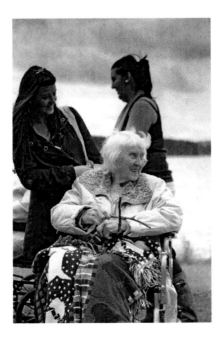

Figure 3.3 Woodland Celebration with the Woodland Trust Scotland

COTTON CONNECTIONS WITH NATURE

We gave participants of the celebration day strips of cotton to record their connections with nature. These were tied to trees and bushes along a loch-side walk and included the following connections and reflections:

'Seeing the natural scenery and different types of plants.'

'Wildlife and plants, loch and bats, swans, cygnets and ducklings.'

'Animal sounds, people laughing, children singing.'

'I loved feeling the sun on my skin for the first time in ages.'

'The children smiling and chatting.'

'Saw lots of people walking their dogs.'

'Trees, blossom, grass.'

'Beauty of the country and wildlife.'

'I like wildlife because it's fascinating.'

'I enjoyed being in the fresh air.'

'Meeting up with other people and walking together.'

'I loved smelling the flowers.'

'Feeling the sun on my face and hearing the wind in the trees.'

'I enjoyed looking over the loch.'

'People are so friendly.'

This woodland celebration day was intentionally created and designed in the format of a family day out, albeit an extended family of nearly 80 people. Integral to this experience was a picnic lunch, which made everyone feel more at home and which triggered memories for some of childhood picnics and fun outdoors. Many people living with dementia in Britain today have experienced life where, over time, there has been an increasing amount of leisure time and opportunity and an increasing focus on nature spaces as spaces for recreation and holiday. By re-connecting people to these experiences through a supported woodland setting, we can enable people to enjoy activity together, be creative outdoors, take exercise and reminisce.

Hands-on sailing holidays

Part of what makes us British is our relationship with the sea, in that we are island people. Again, this relationship with the sea and with sailing in particular is one which is deeply set in our collective cultural identity, which stretches back from times when people made coracles by hand out of wicker and oxhide to the success of our Olympic sailing teams we see today.

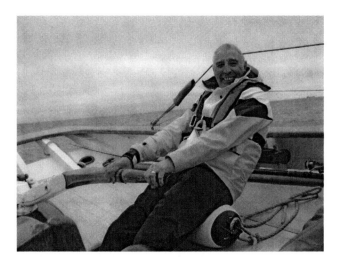

Figure 3.4 Alan Carter sailing in Cornwall

Many people, despite where they live in Britain, feel the pull of the sea and a connection with and a need for coastal vistas and for the salty sea air. For some, their lives have been focused on either working on or around boats and ships or enjoying leisure activities on the water. For me, growing up on a council estate in Essex, sailing for sport and leisure has often been associated with the middle and upper classes. Whilst this association will be familiar for many, there are organisations working hard to break down class stereotypes and increase access to sailing for everyone, including people living with dementia.

Dementia Adventure led two hands-on sailing holidays in 2012, one in Cornwall in partnership with Classic Sailing and one in Essex in partnership with the Sea Change Sailing Trust. John was only 54 when he came on the voyage on the *Eve of St Mawes* in Cornwall with his wife Annie. They both had a marvellous time. John said at the end of the first day, 'I've enjoyed myself, everyone's been happy – no arguments! It's a good day, isn't it?' And at the end of the second day he said, 'We've had such a laugh, and it's cheered me up no end. It's nice to know that there are some very, very kind people out there – they are looking after us.' The sailing adventures involve people living with dementia supported by someone who knows them well actively crewing the boat, steering a course, pulling ropes and sharing the challenge of sailing from A to B over a three- or five-day sail.

Tony is living with dementia and took part in the Essex sailing holiday. He was part of the crew which successfully sailed 92 nautical miles during their group holiday. He said:

> 'I never thought I would have such a chance and I have learnt so much from being on deck with the experienced crew. The sailing was excellent – it was all great.'

Sam and Ben (his sons) said:

> 'What a week and what a team! It was brilliant to meet everyone, to see the beautiful river estuaries, to survive a day of rough seas and high winds, to keep laughing and to learn about the boat and its history. Above all it was so good to see Dad joining in and gaining confidence day by day.'

Christopher (living with dementia) said:

> 'It was a great experience which others should do…it was fun and the people were charming, and the food was good!'

Other feedback we received from family members included:

> 'He has been very positive since coming back from the trip: more positive and animated and with it. Thank you.'

Concluding thoughts

People living with dementia face many challenges during their journey with dementia. At each stage and step of this journey contact and connection with nature presents opportunities for a good quality of life. It presents opportunities to maintain connections with the people and places we love, to enjoy purposeful activity which is good for our wellbeing, and presents opportunities which can be sensitively tailored to our personal and cultural needs and can ultimately lead to people thriving instead of simply surviving. We have highlighted how park walks, woodland experiences and sailing adventures are all linked in with our British cultural identity. Whether it is these activities out in nature, simply sitting on a bench enjoying the morning sun or sitting beside a roaring log fire, by enabling people living with dementia to re-connect with nature we are enabling them to re-connect with living.

Connecting with Dementia Adventure

Dementia Adventure is a multi-award-winning social enterprise specialising in connecting people living with dementia with nature and a sense of adventure. Dementia Adventure is based in Essex but works nationally and has an international following. We provide training, research and consultancy services – all with nature in mind. Income from these activities, donations and grant funding means we can provide award-winning Dementia Adventures from park walks to woodland days out to sailing holidays. Since founding Dementia Adventure in 2009 with Lucy Harding, Neil Mapes and Dementia Adventure have been recognised with a succession of awards, including an International Dementia Excellence Award.

The park walks, woodland celebration days and sailing holidays are all available as films via our YouTube channel. Please watch and share these films. You can find more information at www.dementiaadventure.co.uk or you can follow us on Twitter, become a friend on Facebook and share your own adventures. Do you have an adventure in mind? Call us to discuss it on 01245 230 661.

On Aran

PATRICK BRENCHLEY[1]

At times I've gone across
over to the Aran islands
but not commonly.
I don't come from there.

My brother goes out there
…he's a big man anyway.
He's very taken with them
so he goes back often.

I think it may have been
my brother taking me
in a boat…he's competent…
a strong, strong man.

Once you're out there
I know it really well.
It's a chilly place
but I have a warm feeling about it.

The people are good, but
during the day they somehow slip away.
They've gone, have other places to go to,
but they're still there, they still belong.

The way of life can be attractive
but in a simple way.
It's good in its rights now.
It'll stay. They can do it.

---

1 Poem reproduced from John Killick (ed.) (2010) *The Elephant in the Room: Poems by People with Memory Loss in Cambridgeshire.* Cambridge: Cambridgeshire City Council.

Up to a point
but not all of the time
the scenes come back to me
strongly and with great pleasure.

Chapter 4

Some Southern African Understandings of Nature

MARGARET-ANNE TIBBS

Introduction

In order to understand the importance of nature to people with dementia in southern Africa I felt it was important initially to explore attitudes to nature within the majority black culture. I was able to do this through in-depth discussions with a small sample of women who are well known to me. All except one are now living in the UK. All are familiar with people with dementia, either through their work or from personal experience. They are all black and come from various countries in the region.

Historical and social context

Black African people from this region belong to a single ethnic group called the Bantu, who speak a variety of Bantu languages. The fact that they inhabit different countries and therefore are now of different nationalities is an accident of recent history.

The late nineteenth century saw a race between the various European powers for African land once gold, diamonds and other valuable minerals had been discovered there. Having laid claim to the land, maps were speedily drawn by the winners of the race – meaning that people who were closely related in terms of language and culture sometimes found themselves as inhabitants of different countries. Some of the Nguni people who had moved down the East Coast of southern Africa in previous centuries became first Rhodesians (Southern and Northern) and then Zimbabweans. Others became South Africans.

South Africa itself lies at the southern tip of the African continent, bordered by Namibia, Mozambique, Lesotho, Zimbabwe and

Swaziland. It is a vast country of approximately 471,500 square miles with a population of 50.5 million, of which 79.5 per cent are of black African heritage. The diversity of the population is reflected in the fact that it has 11 official languages, only two of which are of European origin – Afrikaans (evolved from Dutch) and English. As already mentioned, the arbitrary nature of the Colonial map means the languages are not confined to neat geographical boundaries. Most non-English-speaking southern Africans speak several languages. Afrikaans is the language of the descendants of the Boers who trekked away from the British Cape Colony and is spoken by the Afrikaners. But today many Afrikaans speakers are people of mixed race.

It is this extraordinary ethnic and lingual complexity which led Archbishop Desmond Tutu to coin the phrase 'the Rainbow People of God'.

The Rainbow People find themselves now, post-1994 – in what people are now calling the 'post-Mandela' years – facing many challenges. While many have a far higher standard of living than their parents, about a quarter of the population is unemployed and lives on less than $1.25 a day. In some areas such as Gauteng (formerly the Transvaal) a culture of violent crime linked to theft has developed. As well as the terrible legacy of 40 years of apartheid this is also probably a symptom of the fact that South Africa is ranked in the highest ten countries of the world for income inequality. People with enough money living next door to people almost without money leads to shanty towns near gated communities, security guards, armed response teams and many, many guns.

The various medical conditions such as HIV/Aids, TB and malaria pose daunting challenges of course. There are many child- and granny-led households where all the adults of working age have died from sickness.

The central importance of the family

The family unit is large, and nowadays is often geographically spread out. It includes different generations and even reaches beyond the grave to the ancestors. The family name is all-important, and much effort is directed towards upholding and improving its reputation. Many of the elders prefer to live in the rural areas. Families will take them with them when they move to the towns, but the elders do not remain there. They are clearly very unhappy and this dilemma is hard for the family to solve. The elders want to return to the old house and they dearly wish to die there and be buried near their ancestors. They will contentedly help to prepare the food, tend the garden or do traditional craftwork. They are always busy. Everybody understands and accepts this desire, and it works well until the elders become mentally and/or physically frail.

One of my respondents told me about her grandfather – born in 1926 – who 'you will never find inside the house. He spends every day visiting neighbours – and because each village is always some distance from the next, he may walk many miles each day.'

The importance of the ancestors

Veneration of the ancestors as a belief system appears to be widespread in Africa. At its summit is a belief in a Supreme Being who can only be approached by the ancestors. When a person dies, their spirit remains in the homestead – a benign protection for their descendants. This gives the village a spiritual meaning beyond that of the family home. Traditional healers can talk to the ancestors directly but they are not able to speak to the Supreme Being. Southern Africa did not meet with Christianity until the missionaries arrived in the mid-nineteenth century, and it is perhaps surprising how easily traditional religion adapted to Christianity. The major Christian denominations were involved from very early times in education and medical projects, which were of clear benefit to the community. Most Christians, including those in positions of leadership – now largely black – find ways to accommodate the traditional belief system.

Black southern African culture is based on the premise that people want to be together. We have seen this working out through the hierarchy of the family, including the dead with the living. The worst possible thing that could happen to you – worse than death because, after all, ancestors survive in spirit though not in body – would be to be expelled from your family group. Nobody wants to be alone.

Attitudes towards elders

Respect for the living elders is a central plank of African society. It transcends changes in life circumstances. As Nombulelo told me:

> They are an important point of reference for us. In anything we seek or do we have to include the elders, even if they have dementia. We believe that their souls embrace us and give direction, no matter how old they are; their blessing reaches for a long way. So they are never going to be ignored. If we cannot hold a conversation with them we still behave with respect. You would never ignore them, just as you would never ignore the demands your children are making on you... Africans measure their wealth by the pleasure they derive from their families, which in turn are part of the communities – of which the ancestors are a part. If you treat your parent with dementia well it means you acknowledge them; you know they made you no matter what state they are living in now.

The importance of the homestead

Annie and Beulah (Zimbabweans) explained to me that the family/ ancestral home has tremendous importance. Straight away we come across a problem with language. For me those two phrases are interchangeable. For them, the home is where the family lives but, very importantly, it is also where the ancestors live.

The homestead is a microcosm of the land itself:

> It will be heavily guarded because people want to guard their landscape as well as their possessions. A typical African village home will have some sort of orchard with mangoes, guavas, peaches, etc. It will have an area of land surrounding the orchard, depending on the type of land. This is kept as wild as possible: trees, big rocks and wild fruits are usually preserved in their natural state to act as a further level of protection. There also are domestic animals such as dogs, chickens, goats, etc. roaming around. Nearby there will be kraals, usually constructed of thorn branches, in which the cattle and goats are kept safe. Outside the homesteads the fields are ploughed in contours to prevent erosion from the heavy rains and also to divide the

crops into different areas. During the rainy season the landscape may become very beautiful, especially if there is water nearby, and this is the most prized area of the homestead. This is where visitors will be taken before they all settle down to entertain. But as long as the weather is good all the main activities of the household happen outside.

(Annie)

If I, as a white woman, ask a Zulu/Xhosa speaker where they live they will often give the area where 'ekhaya' (homestead) is situated even if they are now living in a town.

Increasingly, as people leave their homesteads for the towns, these family/ancestral homes fall into disrepair. However, some families still return to the ruined homestead to preserve it. All they do is build a slightly more modern house, sink a bore hole, install some solar powered energy, and build some decent lavatories. However, the original thatched hut kitchen will be preserved as it was – repaired rather than rebuilt. At this stage it is used as a holiday home and will only be visited about four or five times a year, especially at Christmas.

(Nombulelo)

As I have said, the relationship between black southern Africans and the landscape they inhabit is very different to that of the white people. The individual belongs to the landscape.

The relationships between the elders and the homestead

As we have seen, the pull for the elders to return to the family ancestral home is very strong:

They want to return to the peace and beauty of the bush and they want to be near the ancestors, which gives them a great peace of mind. They like to feel close to the people who have gone before them. They mostly wish to be buried with their ancestors as well. Not only have they returned to the community, they are finally surrounded by beautiful scenes away from the crowded towns.

(Beulah)

The relationship with the land

The relationship between black southern Africans and the land they inhabit is very different from that with which we are most familiar in this country. This part of the world has to be one of the most beautiful on the planet and yet, on the whole, black southern Africans do not go out especially to see it. Beulah, a Zimbabwean woman I spoke to about this, said, 'Come to think of it, I have never been to the Victoria Falls and I don't know anybody who has!' Gab'sile, from Swaziland, adds: 'We see warthogs and crocodiles in the bush and lots of snakes. They are dangerous. Why would we bother to see them in a game reserve?'

White South Africans, on the other hand, often have a profound and spiritual love for the beauties of their homeland – a fact which has been used to develop the booming South African tourist industry. This may well be an emotional strategy to help them come to terms with the loss of social and economic, as well as political, power which has happened since 1994. These are the people and their children who, growing up, benefited from apartheid, and those who have remained in South Africa are in the process of making some very painful transitions. The beauties of the landscape and the wonders of the wildlife probably provide some degree of solace.

Understanding dementia

As we have seen, the elders are treated with great respect and are of central importance to their culture. Here again the different world view can be shown when making comparisons between cultures.

Nombulelo, with whom I have been corresponding, made a remark which belongs to her culture – not to mine. 'He [her father] is travelling back to his childhood in his mind… I applaud all the good things he has done,' she said, 'but with my dad I had to accept and allow him to age.' I take this to mean that she has to allow him to journey closer to his ancestors (including his wife).

An afterthought on this subject: this family are very strong and committed members of one of the mainstream Christian denominations – but they do not have any problems accommodating their belief system with that of veneration of the ancestors. The two belief systems are generally able to accommodate each other.

In the case of people with dementia in families which may be called 'Western', the medical model is very much the dominant one. This fits easily with the view that loss of cognitive abilities is an indicator that the person is – on one level – travelling back in time to childhood. With families of a traditional African world view, the story may be darker. It may be believed that a spell has been placed upon the person and a visit to the Sangoma (the traditional healer who has an extensive knowledge of the medicinal herbal remedies and cures) is needed.

In neither narrative would the family be familiar with the word 'dementia'. It is understood either as part of the normal ageing process or as the person being cursed. It is only through Western education that people have learned about this illness called dementia. Several people with whom I talked said that it was only when they attended training courses as part of their work that they learned of dementia and began to understand that it is an illness.

The picture I have gradually built up is of individuals who are part of a closely knit landscape. The bush in which they live is so essential to who they are that is almost impossible for them to imagine life away from it. As people age, the need to return to the particular landscape which contains their homestead becomes hard to resist. For people with dementia this need to be enfolded by the landscape may become essential to their wellbeing.

Cross-cultural misunderstandings

It is not surprising therefore if we sometimes find a judgemental attitude by care workers from southern Africa towards the practice in the UK of moving the elders to live in care homes when they become physically and/or mentally frail and dependent. This feeling is not openly discussed with members of the dominant culture – unless there is a high degree of trust. The custom of allowing residents in care homes to spend hours at a time in their room is viewed with disfavour. The fact that this may be an expression of personal choice is treated with manifest disbelief – as are expressions such as 'An Englishman's home is his castle' or the proud statement that 'I have always kept myself to myself'. It is just not believable to them that people would be on their own from choice.

The fact that a way of showing respect for the elders is to avoid making eye contact can easily be shown to be problematic. A black care worker from southern Africa will naturally feel great respect for an older person, even if they are disabled. But they will show respect by not making direct eye contact with them. The person with dementia sees a black worker failing to make eye contact with her and immediately assumes she is not to be trusted.

Apart from one person I spoke to, all my respondents are well known to me. Nombulelo, living in Gauteng, took great pains with email responses to my questions. I hope it gave her a framework to talk through her feelings about her mother, my close friend, as well as her father who is living with dementia. But all the others, working in social care in the UK, were aware of what my attitudes would be towards a view of dementia as a 'second childhood'. Nevertheless, in unguarded moments these attitudes were expressed.

There is clearly major work to be done in providing cultural awareness training for them because their narrative of dementia care, grounded within the family, the homestead, the village and the ancestors, simply does not fit easily into current UK majority culture:

> When we were small children we would come back to the house in the village, after walking miles home from school. The first person we would rush to was Granny. She would be sitting outside on her mat, in the shade, and she would always have time to talk to us. She was mentally confused and I understand now that she may have had dementia. But she would always be busy – preparing food, maybe making traditional crafts. She would never be alone. She was outside because that was where she wanted to be. I think she liked to look at the veld all around her.
>
> (Gab'sile)

This may be an idealised memory but it is an archetype which is firmly believed by black southern Africans. In a part of their world where sunshine is predictable and rainfall is also not only predictable but very desirable, all the major activities of the family/ancestral home take place outside within the landscape. This is normality. I can see that the relationship between human beings and landscape – with or without dementia – is profoundly important, and this differs profoundly in various countries and cultures. The idea of meaningful activities taking place outside as part of an accepting and supportive group is a very beguiling one. How can we adapt this to a climate like that of the UK? Can we make more creative use of indoor spaces to produce the sense of light and fresh air? Can we have plants growing inside as they used to do in Edwardian conservatories?

Because we have many people in the UK working in the field of social care who come from other parts of the world, including southern Africa, we need to learn how to take the best from other cultures in order to improve the quality of dementia care in this country. We also need to educate ourselves about these deeply held cultural values which govern how people behave. No amount of training about best practice will be effective until we can find a way to create a dialogue which can articulate the values and beliefs held by the oldest generation in this country as well as understanding the values and beliefs of workers from other countries. Simply teaching staff techniques to improve care can never be enough unless we also find a way to do this.

Chapter 5

Contact with the Natural World within Hospital Care

SARAH WALLER AND ABIGAIL MASTERSON

Introduction

Many people with dementia will have contact with hospital environments, be they acute hospitals, community hospitals or mental health facilities. Indeed, at any one time estimates suggest that more than a quarter of all acute hospital patients will have a degree of cognitive impairment. Hospitals, like all organisations, have their own particular cultures, and the importance of the right organisational culture in ensuring a positive experience of care for older people has frequently been emphasised. For example, at the beginning of this century a key aim of the National Service Framework (NSF) for Older People in England (Department of Health 2001) was promoting 'culture change so that all older people and their carers are always treated with respect, dignity and fairness'. More recently, organisations such as Alzheimer's Society have highlighted the detrimental effect of hospital stays on the wellbeing and independence of people with dementia (Alzheimer's Society 2009). The physical environment has a demonstrable impact on culture. The King's Fund's Enhancing the Healing Environment (EHE) programme, which began in 2000, aims to encourage and enable local teams to work in partnership with service users and their relatives to improve the physical environment of care. In this chapter we draw on the experience and insights gained from the EHE programme as a whole as well as the 26 schemes in a variety of sites across England that have particularly involved the active use of nature in developing supportive environments for people with dementia.

Hospital environments and people with dementia

Going into hospital is a potentially frightening and bewildering experience for anyone, and for people with dementia the unfamiliar surroundings, noise and very busy spaces pose particular challenges. People with dementia are generally, though not always, older people, who may already have poorer sight and hearing. The impact of this on their ability to make sense of their environment is likely to be exacerbated by the disturbance to their orientation and cognitive processes caused by their dementia. Consequently, people with dementia are likely to:

- be confused and agitated in hospital environments, particularly if they are visually over-stimulated, for example with a plethora of signs and notices

- be unable to see things, for example handrails and toilet seats, if these are the same colour as the wall or sanitary-ware

- experience shadows or dark strips in flooring as a change of level and therefore try to step over them

- resist walking on shiny floors as they may think they are wet

- want to explore and walk around.

However, if hospital environments are appropriately designed it is possible to reduce confusion and agitation, encourage independence and social interaction, and enable people with dementia to retain their ability to undertake activities of daily living.

Florence Nightingale (1859) understood the importance of a well-designed hospital environment:

> Little as we know about the way in which we are affected by form, colour, by light, we do know this, that they have a physical effect. Variety of form and brilliancy of colour in the objects presented to patients is the actual means of recovery.

She also advocated the health-giving properties of access to fresh air and light. More recently the seminal work of Roger Ulrich in the USA in the 1980s, which has been built on since by researchers across the globe, has demonstrated through rigorous scientific studies that enabling access to nature has a positive impact on patients' wellbeing and influences patient outcomes such as reducing anxiety, lowering blood pressure and lessening pain (Ulrich 1984). Conversely, research has also linked poor design and unsupportive environments to negative effects such as delirium, depression, pain and longer hospital stays (Davis, Fleming and Marshall 2009).

Enhancing the Healing Environment programme

Patients are at the centre of The King's Fund's Enhancing the Healing Environment (EHE) programme. The programme was launched in 2000 with the aim of encouraging and enabling local teams to work in partnership with service users to improve the environment of care for all patients in general hospitals. Since then, different waves of the programme have had different foci. For example, in 2008 the focus was improving the environment of care for patients receiving palliative care, their relatives and the bereaved as part of the Department of Health's work to support implementation of the National End of Life Care Strategy; and then in 2009 the focus changed to environments for people with dementia in acute hospitals and mental health settings. Since its inception, over 230 teams from acute, community and mental health NHS trusts, hospices and the prisons service have developed local schemes which have not only transformed the physical care environment but have also supported service change and innovation.

Evaluations of the EHE programme have highlighted the success of the programme in bringing a sense of 'normality' to the hospital environment – for example, by:

- creating a sense of welcome and reassurance on arrival

- developing garden retreats to provide a contrast to the pressurised internal space of the hospital

- designing social spaces that provide a dignified and comfortable space for meeting relatives and friends away from the clinical environment.

Each of these characteristics goes towards creating a more therapeutic and supportive environment for all patients, but they also provide a base from which to explore the additional features that can better support people with dementia in hospitals.

Developing Supportive Environments of Care for People with Dementia programme

The latest phase of the EHE programme has focused on developing more supportive design for people with dementia in hospital. It became clear, during this programme, that many staff had little understanding of the effect of the environment on people with dementia:

> Despite my background as a dementia nurse, I have to admit that I had very little understanding at the start of the project of how the environment can affect people with dementia. This has been the greatest lesson and now I am equipped with the evidence and ability to highlight the benefit to others.
>
> (Dementia Specialist Nurse – EHE team member)

Many carers, on the other hand, were able to describe the most important aspects of the environment that would help lessen anxiety and distress:

> The use of light, more spacious areas and being able to go outside, from my experience as a carer, these were the main things needed to help with lessening aggression and irritability.
>
> (Carer – EHE team member)

The fundamental importance of nature

A recurring theme throughout the different phases and 230 environmental transformation projects supported by the EHE programme since 2000 has been the fundamental importance of access to nature in promoting wellbeing in healthcare environments. Creating links to nature and the natural world, whether by creating outside spaces for people to enjoy or by 'bringing the outside in' by using natural materials and colours and by introducing artworks that reflect the landscape, has repeatedly been demonstrated as having a positive effect on patients and their families as well as staff.

The theory of anthroposophy is described in Chapter 9, and multiple research studies have consistently indicated that simply viewing nature can produce significant recovery or restoration from stress. Even acutely stressed patients can experience a significant reduction in stress levels after only a few minutes of looking at natural settings with greenery, flowers or water and/or looking at representational art depicting serene, natural, open spaces.

As part of the education that is at the heart of the EHE programme, multi-disciplinary teams, which include a patient or carer as a peer alongside clinical and estates professionals, are asked to rate a series of photographs of healthcare settings as Good, Bad or Ugly. Consistently, no matter the focus of the particular healthcare area being reviewed, photographs of parks, gardens, rivers, outside spaces and landscape artworks are classed in the Good category.

Furthermore, consultations undertaken as part of a phase of the EHE programme particularly focused on improving environments for palliative care patients consistently showed that links to nature and the natural world were extremely important for people at the end of their lives and their visitors. Views of nature and/or being able to go outside were highly valued, as were the use of natural materials and the incorporation of the elements, internal planting and the use of artworks depicting nature in interior designs.

Incorporating nature in the hospital environment

Twenty-six schemes which sought to either improve outside spaces or to bring some elements of the outside in have been completed as part of the recent EHE programme to improve the care of people with dementia in hospital settings. Of these, five involved the creation or re-design of gardens so that people with dementia and their carers could have safe, open access to the outside and engage in meaningful activity such as looking after the planting. A palliative care suite for people with dementia also included the development of a private garden into which the patient's bed could be pushed.

Patients with dementia have been actively encouraged to contribute to the individual schemes, and many innovative ways of enabling and supporting their involvement have been developed, for example using coloured cards and paint charts to inform planting and colour choice, participatory arts events such as making a mosaic, and poetry workshops. A universal request from patients and carers is to include a water feature in the design. This has sometimes challenged hospitals where health and safety concerns have been raised initially, but the teams have managed to overcome such objections by emphasising the likely therapeutic impact.

The garden schemes have varied in size and scope depending on the available space. There have been very positive comments from patients, relatives and staff about the use of rubberised materials for pathways, which make walking easier and provide an excellent surface for wheelchairs. A particularly innovative scheme involved the creation of a small garden from two parking spaces adjacent to an acute ward. Initial concerns regarding the size of the garden have been confounded with the design maximising every inch – there is even enough space for patients to engage in outdoor activities such as skittles, offering much fun and great diversion during the summer.

For two schemes, both located on the first floor of hospital buildings, the projects involved the design and construction of robust balcony gardens with adjoining social spaces so that people could enjoy looking at the garden even in inclement weather. Even in these small spaces, principles of good design for people with dementia such as providing returning pathways, interesting but safe planting in raised beds, shelter from sun and rain and a choice of seating have been adhered to.

Evaluation of these garden schemes is ongoing, but early indications are that they are providing calm but interesting areas where people can get away from the pressured hospital wards to enjoy gardening activities, walking, or just sitting and looking at the flowers and planting. Patients are gaining great pleasure from the outside spaces at all times of the year and the direct connection with nature, feeling the wind and the rain, in all weathers. Staff report that access to natural light is helping orientation, and involvement in activities seems to be helping people keep awake during the day and sleep better at night.

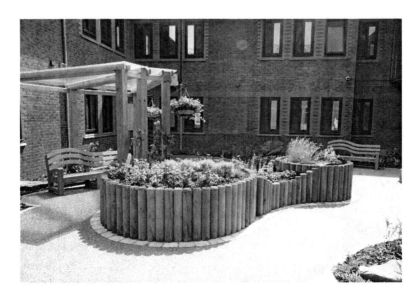

Figure 5.1 Garden areas enable direct connection with nature

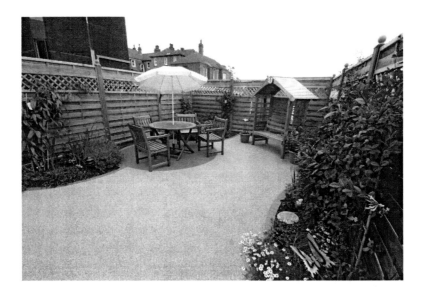

Figure 5.2 Garden areas enable direct connection with nature

All the schemes in wards have focused on making what can be strange, stark, cluttered and confusing spaces more understandable and helping people with dementia to find their way around. Colour and contrast have been used to differentiate bed bays, which can look very similar, and bed spaces have been signposted using images or memory boxes. Wherever possible the re-designs have sought to bring a sense of familiarity to the hospital environment, for example by making sure chairs in social spaces are grouped in small clusters, as people would experience at home, creating domestic-scale dining areas and by using traditional and recognisable sanitary-ware in bathrooms and toilets.

Reinforcing the case for the universal interest in nature, the overwhelming choice amongst patients, carers and staff for images to help orientation and recognition has been flowers, often combined with colour – for example, daffodils with yellow accent walls or poppies with red accent walls. Some hospitals have specially commissioned floral artworks to go around doorways and over bed heads while others have used photographs of flowers. The flowers have been extremely successful in helping people recognise their bed bays and individual bed spaces as well as producing an aura of calm and wellbeing – one patient, when looking at the flowers, even remarking that the ward smelt nice.

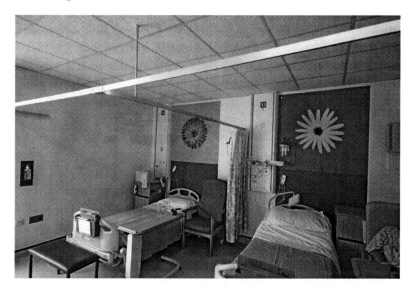

Figure 5.3 Flowers help people recognise their bed space

Light boxes have been used in many areas where there is little natural light. These have the added advantage of staff being able to change landscape photographs to reflect the seasons, acting as an aid to orientation. Larger images of gardens have been placed behind reception desks, and images of woodlands have been printed onto wallpaper, used from floor to ceiling, to give a welcoming first impression of wards. The feedback on the use of this type of floor-to-ceiling image has been overwhelmingly positive and has created a very welcoming and calming entrance to a busy ward.

'Is your ward dementia-friendly?' An assessment tool

As an outcome from the programme, carers have been instrumental in the development of an assessment tool called 'Is your ward dementia-friendly?' (available at www.kingsfund.org.uk/projects/enhancing-healing-environment/ehe-design-dementia). This practical, easy-to-use tool has been informed by evidence and best practice and designed for use by carers together with staff to assess the ward environment. There are a number of questions that specifically relate to natural light, views of nature and access to outside spaces because these have proved to be such key elements in the success of the projects. Extensive testing has indicated that the tool provides a useful benchmark to measure progress against, as well as a valuable framework for drawing up an action plan for improvement, prompting discussions about both care delivery and the physical environment.

Overarching design principles

The experience from the EHE programme has led The King's Fund to develop overarching design principles which bring together best practice in creating more supportive care environments for people with cognitive problems and dementia. The principles were drawn from a number of sources, were informed by research evidence and are grouped around the desired outcomes for people with dementia in ward environments. These outcomes are easing decision making; reducing agitation and distress; encouraging independence and social interaction; promoting safety; and enabling activities of daily living. Although developed for use initially in hospitals, the design principles have potential for use in all health and social care settings and even in the home environment.

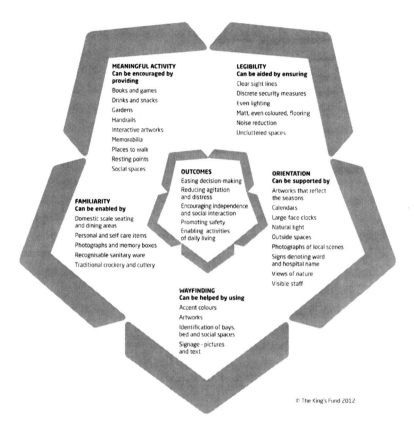

Figure 5.4 Developing supportive design for people with dementia: Overarching design principles

Outside spaces, gardens, views of nature and artworks that reflect the seasons are all important elements identified in the principles.

Rising to the challenge

The schemes, which have been undertaken in mental health and community units and acute trusts, show how relatively straightforward and inexpensive changes to the design and fabric of the care environment can have a considerable impact on the wellbeing of people with dementia. The EHE programme has demonstrated how appropriately designed environments have the potential to reduce the incidence of agitation and challenging behaviour and the prescription of anti-psychotic medication, promote independence, improve nutrition and hydration, increase engagement in meaningful activities and encourage greater carer involvement as well as improving staff morale, recruitment and retention, all of which contribute to a reduction in overall service costs (Waller, Masterson and Finn 2013).

Sceptics might assume that improving the appearance and usability of an area must be an expensive, time-consuming activity and a luxury that the NHS cannot afford in the current economic climate, but providers of healthcare services will continue to need to maintain and improve the buildings in which they deliver care. Experience has shown that incorporation of these design principles need not make refurbishments any more costly. Indeed, using the physical environment as a focus to build the thought and understanding of staff locally about the needs of people with dementia has also had additional benefits in encouraging staff to challenge the norm more generally on behalf of patients.

Better physical environments of care are also better places to work in and make staff feel more valued. Extensive consultation and engagement with service users and their relatives and friends is at the core of the EHE programme and results in significant changes to the organisational culture and staff 'owning' and taking responsibility for their work environment. Staff are supported to develop a range of skills during their participation in EHE, including the ability to constructively challenge organisational norms if they believe this is right for their patients. The teams are rightly very proud of their achievements and many carers have gained great support and really valued the opportunity to use their knowledge for the benefit of others. For staff, the opportunity to work so closely with people with dementia and their carers has enabled them to develop an improved understanding of dementia and how best to support their patients in hospital:

> EHE has turned my practice around! I am much more confident and articulate. Work is a pleasure every day and I have become absolutely passionate about the needs of people with dementia.
>
> (EHE team member)

Chapter 6

How Norwegian People with Dementia Experience Nature

SIDSEL BJØRNEBY

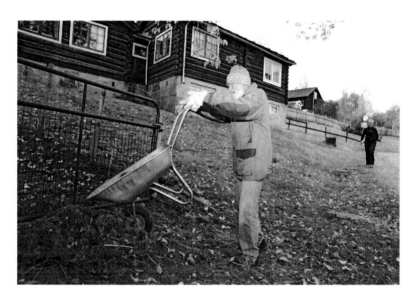

Figure 6.1 Trond shows how he enjoys helping with outdoor activities in Vaagaa, 2013
Source: Ketil Sandviken and GD

Our country – Norway – has a long and varied coastline, sometimes steep and sometimes with a small coastal strip, and a mountainous inland. Traditionally, nature represents what we value in Norway. Even though the population is becoming more and more urban, most old persons in cities have spent their childhood and youth in rural districts, where life was close to and dependent on nature.

Care staff are often young, and a growing number have a background from countries far away. Therefore they are seldom familiar with the kind of childhood experiences that older people have. Today young people often have different interests from that which is represented by life on farms. Urban life is considered by many to be more desirable.

One nurse from Sri Lanka told me: 'I have no idea what Mrs A talks about when she talks about her childhood and parents. Is there some literature where I can learn more about old times in Norway?' I suggested that she should ask Mrs A's son if he could share some information about this. She did, and became so interested that she wanted to go to the library to find out more. It is a good activity for the relatives of people with dementia to share photos and stories with the staff, and in some way try to explain their backgrounds. But this is also necessary for the staff if they are going to use such knowledge when planning activities and trips for older people with backgrounds that differ from their own.

Two aspects of Norwegian nature are particularly relevant for the memories of the old days. Probably Norwegian people's love and appreciation of nature can be due to these aspects. These aspects are life on the coast and life on farms.

Life on the coast

In earlier times, fishing was the main livelihood. Fathers went out fishing in harsh weather, or were away as seamen. Children had to get to school by boat. Fish was the main food, and sometimes there could be quite poor living conditions. Still, even today, the open sea, coastal landscape and a feeling of fresh air and freedom are worshipped and sources for fond reminiscence when they are seen in retrospect.

Nowadays the homes along the fjords and by the coast are often used as vacation homes in the summer by children or grandchildren of the fishermen or sailors who lived there 50 or 100 years ago. In the winter these former homes are often deserted. It is difficult to imagine the hardship experienced in the long and dark winters with short days and long and dark nights, and maybe no electricity.

Life on farms

Many small farms were owned by the farmers themselves, with maybe five to ten cows, a horse, some sheep and goats or maybe a couple of pigs and some chickens, and were self-sustaining households. This was normal up to 50–60 years ago. Children took part in all the work on the farm.

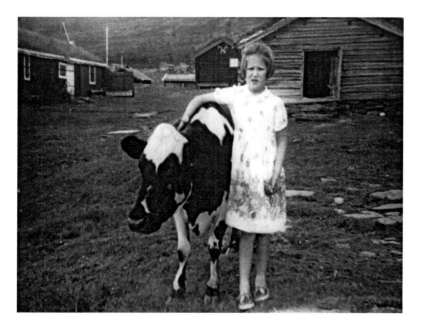

Figure 6.2 Randi loved her cows, 1958

Many children only went to school for three days a week. Because of this, they were natural contributors to the household and farming activities, and were expected to take over the farm sooner or later. The work in the winter might be feeding the animals, milking, cleaning and mending clothes. In the summer and autumn, work might consist of cultivating vegetables, harvesting the hay and grain or picking potatoes.

One day at a nursing home where the occupational therapist organises different activities in their outside space, a man with dementia said while sawing wood, 'It's so good to be out in the countryside again!'[1] Obviously the activity of wood-sawing brought back some good memories. In care homes the staff often find it difficult to give people with dementia activities that make them feel even a bit useful. A lady in the same care home who had

1   Occupational therapist Anne Moseby, Manglerudhjemmet, Oslo.

grave cognitive problems and rarely spoke suddenly became aware of a large dandelion and exclaimed, 'I just need to take this up.' It provided a useful basis for a meaningful conversation about how she had worked outdoors in her earlier life.

Seters

From farms the cattle were herded and walked up to the mountains above the tree line to small temporary summer farms called 'seters' at the end of June. The hay at the main farm in the valley needed to be kept for the long winter months, so the animals had to be sent away. Normally a seter would consist of a log cabin for living in, accommodation for the cattle at night and a barn for storing the hay from a small field.

The cattle would go freely into the mountain terrain all day, but return to be milked in the evening. The cows were called by the milk maid, who would call and sing to help them find their way back. These melodies have inspired Norwegian songs and folk music up till today. Recordings of such songs could bring back fond memories.

It was common to produce cheese and butter at the seter, for one's own use. But there was usually no electricity, and water came from a stream close by. Life at the seter was seen as romantic, but it was also quite hard.

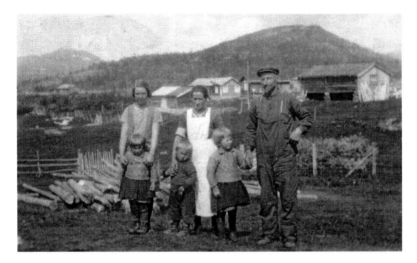

Figure 6.3 The whole family stayed at the seter each summer, 1929

But talking to older people who have experienced this life in the mountains can reveal happy memories. Other older people may have visited the seters and maybe spent the night when hiking in the mountains to enjoy the beauty of the nature. Unlike in many other countries, the seters were actually a part of nature and of the experience when visiting mountain districts.

Today there are very few seters in actual use in the way that they were in earlier times. Automation and changed attitudes to farming life have resulted in many log cabins in the seters being transformed to vacation houses, or cabins (in Norway we call them hyttes), with no animals. They are frequently being used in the winter also.

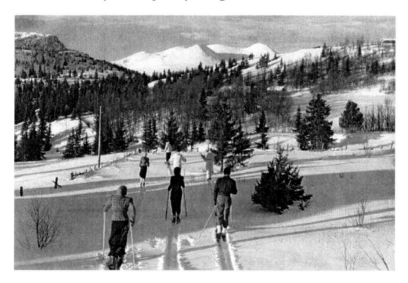

Figure 6.4 Norwegian winter Sunday skiing, 1945

Hyttes

A large proportion of Norwegians have 'hyttes'. They are holiday houses, sometimes in groups, but usually standalone houses. Often they have previously been seters in the mountains, or in the forest, by the fjord or on the coast. Also, newer hyttes or holiday houses have been built in the same areas. These hyttes are today used in summer as well as winter, and even for weekends.

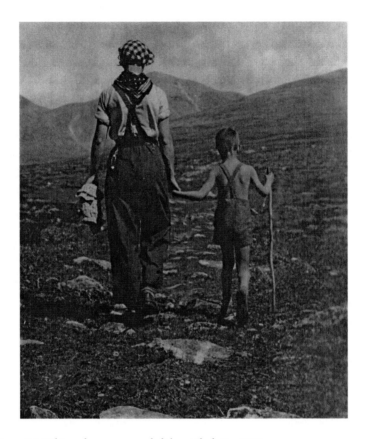

Figure 6.5 Hiking when on summer holiday at the hytte, 1933

Life can be simpler than at home. Generations spend time together, and nature is always close. There are usually no gardens, because the presence and beauty of nature itself feels more relevant.

Many people with dementia have fond memories of life in these hyttes or vacation homes and a life close to nature. They may have a longing for the happy days that they spent as children and young people, and later with families and children of their own.

However, it is not easy to let them have this practical experience as they age. Sometimes there is no access for a car, and possibly no electricity or running water. Care homes are having to be innovative.

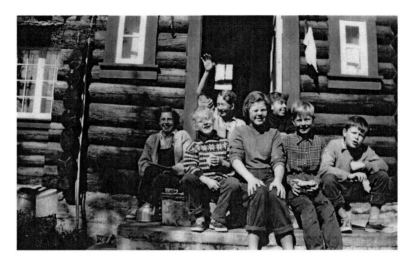

Figure 6.6 Breakfast in the sun at the family hytte, 1956

Care homes and Green Care

Gradually many nursing homes have or are planning gardens or sensory gardens in order to give people with dementia opportunities to enjoy the outdoors with flowers and shrubs. Sometimes there are small ponds, birdbaths and benches, and the possibility of simple gardening activities. Some enjoy just being there and peacefully smell, listen, watch and experience the fresh air. These gardens are valuable, but are of a more urban nature. They are very different from the wild nature that many older people have experienced.

In the winter with scarce daylight and ice and cold, it is difficult for staff in nursing homes to find good outdoor activities. I know of one occupational therapist who sometimes takes a resident for a short skiing trip, but this usually takes more resources than are available.

Would it be possible to let some people with dementia experience wild nature, if this is a happy part of their life? A county in the middle of Norway, Vaagaa, has taken this challenge seriously.[2] They have a centre called 'Green Care', a day-care centre for people with dementia who live at home. (For more information about Green Care for people with dementia, see Chapter 6 of *Transforming the Quality of Life for*

2   Jorunn Heier, project 'Groenn omsorg', Klones, Vaagaa, Norway.

People with Dementia through Contact with the Natural World [Gilliard and Marshall 2011].) Vaagaa is an agricultural community with about 4000 inhabitants. There are large areas of mountains and a rich culture of outdoor life and beautiful old houses. Twice a week a group of persons with dementia, many of them men who have a desire for outdoor activities, meet at a former school for agriculture. They tend to the garden and other outdoor areas, prune fruit tress and bushes, cut grass and chop firewood. They also take part in carpentry, kitchen work and cultural activities.

Most days those staff who have experience and knowledge of the needs of people with dementia will fill up a minibus with 5–6 persons and take day trips. The trips may be to a seter or mountain hut that belongs to the family of one of the participants, to a lake for fishing trout, or to somewhere to pick wild berries. In the winter they may also sometimes go for trips, but generally it is easier in the summer. In addition, they may have activities at the day-care centre, such as making bird-houses or sawing and even chopping wood.

Some quotes from the participants:

> 'The best day I have ever had!' (This from a lady who hardly ever talks.)

> 'Let us walk slowly, I want to be outdoors as long as I can.'

Sometimes they go to the seter or hytte that belongs to the family of one of the users. They find that the older person starts to tell stories about many things from earlier days. They may tell the same stories as they did last time they visited with the group, and the other participants often add remarks as well. It might be about the mountain-tops around, about having been a timber worker, or having made a new roof 40 years earlier on the seter.

This day-care centre is a great success, and could be copied by other rural counties. The day trips clearly bring out positive memories and give people a sense of having had abilities. Family carers find it helpful when a parent or spouse returns home happy and contented.

Other ideas

1. In cities, however, it is not so easy to get access to seters or hyttes. Through contact with local Alzheimer Associations, possibly in co-operation with local Tourist Associations, would it be possible to find some huts in the mountains or the forest or simple houses by the sea that could be used for day trips by small groups of people with dementia? The Norwegian Tourist Association already has trips for seniors, but has not yet thought of seniors with dementia as a target group. The places to visit would have to be similar to what they were like 50–100 years ago, and of course accessible by car or boat.

2. Another idea is to use some of the old hotels that used to be visited by nature-loving people when not everybody had their own hytte or could afford trips abroad. Many of these hotels in the mountains or by the fjords have problems surviving, and are often used as temporary homes for immigrants from Africa or Asia. Maybe some could be used for holidays for people with dementia and their families?

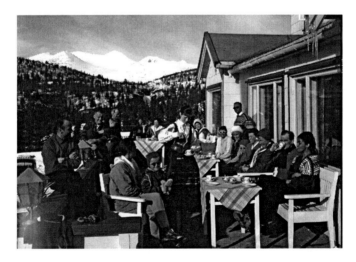

Figure 6.7 This is a typical Easter holiday hotel, showing how the sun is worshipped in the spring, 1961

Such visits would need to be planned carefully, considering the needs of those people with dementia who have a desire to experience nature. Staff would need to be interested in what nature itself means to many older persons. There must be sufficient time and peace to really use and experience the senses, and maybe some tastes of traditional food. To some persons with dementia such trips could bring back just as happy memories as trips to cafés or museums.

3. Another way of bringing memories of nature is using old films and photos from activities on farms or the seter, or life in boats and with fisheries, combined with conversations about the memories of the persons with dementia. However, rushing people with dementia through such experiences could be more harmful than we can comprehend. Allowing people to access memories from their own life requires interest, knowledge and consideration in order to meet their individual needs. And there must be sufficient time to retrieve memories and to talk about them.

Nature itself is sufficient as entertainment – birds singing, mountain streams, the smell of fresh air or the sound and smell of the sea, maybe a taste of wild berries – these are all sensory elements of value and provide a basis for actively bringing out memories and talking about them.

Chapter 7

How People with Dementia Experience Nature in Rural and Island Scottish Communities

GILLEAN MACLEAN

I am a parish minister of the Church of Scotland and have worked in ministry for some 20 years now. I was brought up in a variety of rural situations and trained as a general nurse in Glasgow in the early 1970s. My mother was diagnosed with Vascular Dementia in 2004 and after a short and rather traumatic illness died after a fall while in residential care. It was only after her death and following a post-mortem examination that it was determined that she was in the early stages of Alzheimer's. As an outdoor person, a keen gardener and frequent walker, she had struggled to settle into what was an excellent sheltered housing complex because of the feeling of being 'shut in'. This almost certainly exacerbated her condition. She was found wandering in the street on two occasions with her passport and her walking boots in a bag. She had asked when she moved in if she could help with caring for the complex gardens but was told that these were all landscaped and tended by a firm.

When she was admitted to residential care, again an excellent facility with first-class support and care, which was run by the Church of Scotland, she was given a room with a wonderful view of the hills and trees. She loved the feeling of space and enjoyed her room very much. She enjoyed the company of people she had known in the past when she had played her accordion locally but she still struggled with the inability to get outside. I often asked if she could be taken for a walk in the extensive grounds, but of course this depended on the staffing situation and was not always possible. Her frustration was palpable, and as a family we had explored a variety of options including caring for her at home with a full-time in-house carer. She died suddenly after a fall that could not have been foreseen or prevented after only six weeks in the care home. The difficult decision about her future had been taken out of our hands.

Since that time I have become more and more aware of the rights that we all have to fresh air and outside space and the effect that a denial of this can have on our wellbeing both when we are well and able and, perhaps even more so, when we are unable to care for ourselves.

In my capacity as a minister in a rural island parish off the West Coast of Scotland and now in a rural Aberdeenshire parish, I have had contact over the years with a number of people who have been diagnosed with a variety of age-related illnesses. These are of course wide-ranging, as they are in other groups of our society; however, the Church is one of the agencies that perhaps sees the largest concentration of elderly people on a regular basis and continues to make contact with them and their families during what can be a challenging time. The challenges that they and their families and friends face are similar to those in other parts of the country; however, there are some areas of particular concern for those who live in a rural situation and/or on an island.

The population of the island of Arran fluctuates somewhere around 4500, but a significant number of these people are over retirement age and a further number have travelled to retire on the island from other parts of the country. So, while there is a close island community with many families doing their best to care for their relatives in the home, along with excellent home-care facilities, there are many for whom this is not possible and whose families are some considerable distance away.

The island has a cottage hospital, a private nursing home and a council-run residential home. None of these facilities can meet the needs of all those requiring care, although every effort is made to place as many as possible in one of the local facilities. In preparing this short reflection I have spoken with a number of people diagnosed with dementia and their families. I have asked them to consider the type of care they would wish to have available to them as their condition progresses, thinking particularly of the outdoor space that might be available to them.

The major concern for all has been that they remain on the island that they call home. The horror of being cared for 'off-island' encourages many people to try to manage their problems for as long as they can without intervention. In terms of illness in general, when a choice of receiving treatment involves frequent trips to hospitals on the mainland, many elderly people opt for palliative care that can be provided at home or in the local cottage hospital rather than commit to the stress of travelling and the further possibility of being cared for away from the island.

On two occasions I visited ladies in their eighties who had been very fit and active up until being diagnosed with cancer; both felt they couldn't face the journeys for treatment and opted for palliative care in our local hospital or at home. They were cared for locally with great love and compassion, but their families felt that they had given up too easily and could have had some years of quality living if they had given the treatment a chance. For both of them the thought of being so far from home with few visitors and possibly even dying in a mainland hospital without being able to see the sea was a real and palpable horror. They were afraid that once 'they got you over there' then getting back home to the island would be a struggle.

Following a desire to stay on the island is the thought of not being able to see the sea or the hills. For two of the ladies that I visited, their view of the sea is now the sole topic of conversation. One of these ladies told me that she felt she would not be able to cope if she couldn't see the sea on a daily basis. For 80 years she had lived and worked with the sea as a constant companion and, at a time when familiarity was so important to her wellbeing, it was the sea that remained her constant companion. Another lady, living currently in sheltered housing but with a view of the hills, reminds me on each visit how well she knows the hills that she can see from her window. She is unable to remember the names of her children or her late husband but can tell stories of wandering in the local hills as a child.

A former local midwife agreed to talk to me about her recent diagnosis of Alzheimer's disease and her hopes for her continuing care. I visited her at her home which is situated in a small group of houses surrounded by moors and hills. She told me she was an 'incomer' but had now lived most of her life on the island, and it was her wish to remain in her own home as long as possible. All the doors of the house were open and she told me that she spent a great deal of her time outside, working in the garden, and making sure the birds and other visiting wildlife was fed and watered. She was able to 'ground herself', she said, by watching the changing of the seasons and always looked forward to the arrival of the spring lambs. She couldn't contemplate being cared for in a facility that didn't have access to the outdoors, and if she became unable to walk she felt that at least if she had a view of some kind of wild place and the possibility of watching the birds feeding she would be able to cope.

One gentleman, who has since died, was a keen gardener and had retired with his wife to the island some 20 or so years ago. They had become involved in all aspects of island life and their garden occupied much of their time. The onset of his condition was fairly rapid, and quite quickly following his diagnosis he found himself in our local hospital. He was cared for, for a short time, in our residential facility but was often found to have 'escaped' and was deemed unsuitable for that type of care. In conversation with the gentleman I discovered that it was never his aim to 'escape' – simply to go to collect his newspaper as he had done on a daily basis for over 20 years. Although the facility was providing excellent care, there was no secure outside space where he could potter in the garden nor feel free to walk in safety under supervision. Latterly it was decided that his dementia had reached a stage where his needs could not be met on the island and a facility on the mainland was being sought for his continuing care. This was a source of great distress to him and his wife and it was perhaps providential that his illness escalated rapidly and he died in our own local hospital before any further arrangement could be implemented.

I found it interesting that I was unable to find many people who had worked on the land that had been diagnosed with dementia. This is perhaps a study in itself! I do, however, visit a retired farmer's wife who still lives in her own home and is in the early stages of dementia. From her door she is able to see the ruin of the croft her grandparents farmed and the fields that she worked alongside her late husband. Her family designed the house with large windows, knowing that she would want to be able to see the planting and harvest time and all the daily workings of the farm. For a time after a short physical illness, she stayed with members of her family in the city but became increasingly confused and unable to perform the simplest of tasks. Her anxiety was such that she was unable to settle in the house during the day and spent much of her time walking from room to room.

Her family took her home to her own house on the island for a short time, to allow themselves space to consider more long-term care. However, although returning home was traumatic in itself, they found that she very quickly began to regain the daily living skills she had lost in the city. She told me that her views of the sea and the land surrounding the house helped her on a daily basis to keep in touch with who she was. Currently, appropriate care is being provided to allow her to remain at home. Her family are convinced that it was not simply the unfamiliarity of her accommodation that unsettled her while away from home but her inability to see and experience the round of the seasons and farming life. In her time in the city she lost all track of time and sense of space. Despite being told by professionals that this level of confusion was now permanent and there would be no recovery, her family were amazed at how quickly she became settled and grounded when she returned to the farm. Her ability to deal with dates and days remained impaired but her sense of time and place during the round of 24 hours normalised very quickly.

In my current parish many of the elderly people I visit who have been diagnosed with various types and severity of dementia are from a farming background and have spent their lives in the countryside. Their doors are nearly always open, and access to outside space is a priority for most. There is a horror among all I have spoken to about being 'shut in'. Those who have worked the land or have been involved in animal husbandry take a keen interest in the seasons, and conversations regularly revolve around the state of the weather, the early (or late) lambing season or the accuracy (or lack of it) of the local farmer's ploughing.

With one gentleman who is often unable to remember his surname or the location and number of his family, the conversation is bright with recollections from his working days on the farm. These recollections are usually sparked by the view of worked farmland from his windows. He is able to tell me the type of each crop and the breeding habits and qualities of each animal down to the smallest detail. His everyday living skills are poor and he finds even making a hot drink very challenging, but his ability to give advice to the local younger farmers remains unimpaired. His family are aware of this and, as his daily living skills diminish, they are struggling to see how he would survive in any of the local care homes, however excellent the care. The interest he derives from being able to see the round of farming life is literally keeping his brain alive.

While I am aware that it is not possible to re-create every type of landscape that each person with dementia is familiar with, it seems to me to be literally a matter of life and death to those who have lived their lives in a rural environment that they have access to fresh air and stimulating and familiar views, sounds and smells. Caring for people with dementia is challenging and at times can be frustrating, but the provision of appropriate surroundings and a stimulating environment would benefit the individual themselves, their families and the care staff, allowing for a much more positive experience for all.

Taking to the Hills

JEAN HOWITT[1]

Hills and any parts linked to them
are mine, and totally different shapes.
They are very much to the core here.

What does pull your eyes out
is that there is mountains right across
that are still there to this day.

I had never gone through the life up there,
but I did it, and I had no idea
how certain that background was,

and for the whole part, right down
and right over…it was away for years.
It sweeps on its own feet.

That sweep of country…I suppose
they call it 'Ye Banks and Braes'…
is 'Departed Never to Return', that's

rather sad. But some of the hills
and parts that you have done over time…
they just become part of you.

---

1   Poem reproduced from John Killick (2008) *Dementia Diary: Poems and Prose.*
London: Hawker Publications.

Chapter 8

Digging Up the Roots

Nature and Dementia for First Nation Elders

WENDY HULKO

This chapter addresses the relationship between nature and dementia for Secwepemc Nation Elders,[1] a group of people that views dementia as a relatively new phenomenon brought on largely by colonization and the resulting destruction in their traditional lifestyles. This is not surprising given that one's interconnectedness to and embeddedness within the natural world is integral to Indigenous peoples;[2] the health of the environment is seen to be directly tied to the health of the people, and nature is drawn upon in healing ceremonies performed in sweat lodges and at powwows, for example. Thus, nature has a role to play in the prevention of memory loss in later life and the care of persons with dementia, as will be argued in this chapter.

The quotes in this chapter are drawn from two qualitative research studies undertaken by the author and her colleagues with

---

1   The Secwepemc People are a Canadian First Nation, one of the three groups of Aboriginal peoples in Canada, the others being Inuit and Métis peoples. The traditional territory of the Secwepemc is in the Interior of British Columbia, Canada, and the Nation is made up of 17 communities (www.secwepemc. org/about/ourstory), with populations ranging from 148 to more than 1000 people (http://pse5-esd5.ainc-inac.gc.ca/fnp/Main/Search/TCMain.aspx?TC_NUMBER=1065&lang=eng).

2   'Indigenous' is often used interchangeably with the term 'Aboriginal' in the Canadian context, with the former being more of a global term to indicate the original inhabitants of a particular land mass and the latter being a creation of the Canadian government and a legal designation (see Absolon 2011; Jacklin and Warry 2012).

more than 33 Secwepemc Elders[3] in the Interior of British Columbia, Canada: the first project determined Elders' views on memory loss and memory care in later life and was completed in 2010, including three follow-up interviews on cultural trauma; and the second research project, which ran from 2011 to 2013, aimed to build nursing capacity to care for Elders in a culturally safe way through an educational intervention involving storytelling that was developed in collaboration with Elders. While neither research project focused explicitly on nature, that is, the researchers did not ask about the environment in any of the interviews (Int) or sharing circles (SC), we did collect a fair amount of data on the importance of nature in preventing and responding to dementia. Sharing circles are similar to focus groups in that both of these methods of data collection involve small-group discussions led by a facilitator; however, they are markedly different in that the facilitator of a sharing circle mainly listens and observes and avoids interrupting the participants, plus cultural protocols are followed, including gifting, opening and closing with prayer, acknowledging one's relationship to the land, speaking in turn and listening intently, and ending when the participants determine it is time to end (see Absolon 2011).

For Secwepemc Elders, living within and honouring nature is simply part of being Secwepemc and is encapsulated by the expression 'all my relations', which many Elders – from this and other Nations – say in prayer to the creator. As one male Elder explained:

> When they pray, when [Elders] say 'all my relations', what it really means is that, even in the created, [it] has a little bit of God in it. So all [is] related, what air you breathe or water you drink, it gives you life in your body, it just goes 'round and round'. Those trees out there breathe in what we breathe out, they purify it, and breathe it back in...
>
> (male, SC 4, Oct 2011)

The idea that Indigenous people honour the land and all of the creatures who inhabit it and recognize this interconnectedness is grounded in reality – past and contemporary. That is, while 'the noble

3   Twenty-three Elders participated in the first study and 35 Elders took part in the second. The data in this chapter are drawn mainly from the first study, as the second study was still in progress at the time of writing.

savage' is indeed a harmful stereotype created by non-Indigenous people, this depiction of Indigenous people (as living in the wild and protecting the earth) has its roots in a belief system whose complexity is often mistaken for simplicity. The next section follows on from this introduction to describe aspects of the traditional lifestyle of Secwepemc people and changes brought on by colonization which are thought to have led to dementia.

Traditional lifestyle as preventative

When Elders spoke of the past or 'them days', their words indicated that healthy lifestyles included daily interaction with the natural world and food gathered from the earth. One female Elder told the researchers:

> And I seen [sic] all the trees, the fruit trees that we used to climb [to] get all the fresh berries and Granny used to have goose berries, cherries, apricots, pears. Oh, I remember all that. We used to stand there and hold the basket for Granny when she was up on the ladder picking the fruit.
>
> (female, Int 3, Oct 2010)

Elders in all three communities referenced the gardens, apple orchards, berry picking, deer hunting, meat drying, and fishing that occurred in their childhoods. They explained that:

> long ago we just had our wild meats and…we had vegetables out of our gardens…we ate roots and stuff from the mountains and things like [that].
>
> (female, SC 1, Oct 2008)

Traditional lifestyles also included ceremonies that took place in nature, some of which required the Secwepemc person to spend weeks or months at a time living alone in nature. This is the 'vision quest' – a spiritual ceremony that involves climbing and then staying atop a mountain to await a vision – that another Elder described, noting that more people took part in this process in the past:

> And they went up the mountain to get their spiritual, their annual guidance, spiritual guide. There was [sic] more of them back then. Elders [and other] people tell me it didn't take as

long. Oh yeah, it took longer at that time – because there were so many of them – to get their spiritual help up there on the mountain, their animal spirit. Now, now it's a little harder – two weeks, two months, or more.

(male, Int 2, Oct 2010)

This quote seems to suggest that as Secwepemc people have become more disconnected from nature, their spirituality has suffered. In the past, Secwepemc people were more connected to nature in that their livelihood and spiritual practices were dependent on the health of the environment surrounding them and their accessibility to this natural world. This is no longer the case, as the next section demonstrates.

A changing world

Changes in nature can result in changes in people, and as spiritual practices were forced underground, chemicals were introduced, and food was no longer grown in their communities and/or harvested from the land, these and other changes to traditional lifestyle were implicated in the increasing prevalence of dementia. One Elder pointed to increasing employment and professional careers of family members as a reason for no longer 'living off the land':

All my kids are in some kind of job and they can't – they're not like how it was before like when we lived off the land and hunted and did everything…garden and pick berries and stuff. Now they're employed, they're professionals, and how many professionals could take time off?

(female, Int 1, Feb 2009)

Secwepemc Elders viewed the causes of dementia as largely social and environmental, referencing dietary changes, chemicals, accidents, age, alcohol and drugs, loss of oral culture, medications, pollution, and trauma, including residential schools (Hulko *et al.* 2010, p.327). Causes of dementia that are more environmental than biological and that highlight changing relationships with the natural world have been put forth by members of another BC First Nation dealing with early-onset familial Alzheimer's disease, alongside genetic explanations (Butler *et al.* 2011).

In line with their social-determinants-of-health view of the causes of dementia, the definition of dementia advanced by Secwepemc Elders is more expansive than an issue with 'brain cells', with Elders making reference to 'the tightness in your throat' that comes from not being able to express yourself in your language or 'feeling safe enough to talk about these things on the level that is healing for you and for other people' (female, SC 4, Oct 2011). This is an example of the 'embodiment of oppression' that Neil Henderson (2012) has theorized in relation to Native Americans and dementia. Henderson has posited a model that depicts the ways in which social phenomena convert to physical diseases, with the starting point being genocide, land theft, forced removal, reservations, nutrition trauma, and the colonizer's overall disruption of a sense of coherence for Native Americans, and the end point being white man's stress disease, that is, hypertension, diabetes, and substance abuse.

Henderson argues that the sense of vulnerability and cultural system damage caused by these social phenomena leads to buffering oneself from stress by unhealthy behaviours and interacts with contemporary attacks on sovereignty; and that one's condition worsens over time, with age-associated diseases manifesting. This model of dementia as the embodiment of oppression resonates with Secwepemc views on the causes of dementia and ways to prevent memory loss. 'Bringing back traditional lifestyle' was thought by Secwepemc Elders to be the best way to prevent dementia (Hulko *et al.* 2010), which is akin to returning to a sense of coherence. This bringing back of traditional lifestyle is suggested by the metaphor of 'digging up the roots', which is explained in the section below that addresses nature and storytelling as components of preventing and responding to dementia.

Nature, storytelling, and dementia

The title of this chapter ('Digging Up the Roots') references an actual activity that Elders engage in – now and/or when they were younger – as well as the bringing back of the traditional lifestyle that Elders believe is required in order to prevent dementia (see Hulko *et al.* 2010). Digging in and caring for the earth while telling stories to children is one way Secwepemc Elders work to revive their culture, as explained by the same Elder who shared the meaning of 'all my relations':

> I learned that from [name of Elder], she took me out there, said I need your help, I want to take some roots, and dandelion roots are long, and I went over there, and I started digging and digging, and digging, and it was hard ground. I dug and dug and she has about 20 children gathered around her, and she was telling stories. I dug one out and I handed it to her, and she looked around, 'Oh there is another one out there, go dig that.' But what was happening, it was two things happening: I was digging the root over there which the kids love, but her storytelling to the kids was happening also, and the kids saw me digging up the roots, they saw me come over and show care.
>
> (male, SC 4, Oct 2011)

The preservation and sharing of traditional knowledge was tied to nature, with lessons between Elders and children taking place outside and care for the natural world being demonstrated by Elders. The language was taught and maintained through reference to the environment, and a marker of the loss of language and decrease in memory for one Elder was the failure of youth to recall the names of the mountains surrounding them:

> And so in terms of memory, what I notice is like that even from the little village that I come from, some of the kids are, the teenage kids nowadays, like I ask them, 'Do you know our language? Do you know the names of the mountains that surround us?' And they said no! But they are busy playing with their phone[s] and watching TV and [clears throat], but no language [is] being spoken, and that makes me sad because quite often in our languages you can say a certain word, and that word will cover not just this generation, and my mother's generation, but go down the line back to five, six hundred years ago.
>
> (female, SC 4, Oct 2011)

Another Elder spoke of showing the tomatoes he grows to little kids and letting them dig potatoes in his garden and in the process teaching these young children not only where food comes from, but also that their people were growers in the past and can be in the present:

> I had some Elders visit the greenhouse that we built and they brought a bunch of little kids, and well the little kids, they never saw tomatoes like that, hanging from the roof, eh? Twelve feet high. And then we went to the garden and we dug potatoes and one little boy said, 'What is that doing down there?' He thought potatoes just – these are little kids, like we're growers, originally our people are growers. And the kids couldn't believe this, so they're in there digging the potatoes, running all over the garden, they had more fun then – but you know what really hit me, they thought potatoes come from Safeway, they thought tomatoes come from Safeway [general laughter].
>
> (male, SC 1, Feb 2009)

These two examples of bringing together nature and storytelling in interactions between Secwepemc Elders and children show how practices such as this can foster intergenerational communication, preserve historical and socio-geographic knowledge, and also ensure that Elders maintain an active role in their communities and maintain their brain health. Inter-generational communication such as this is also a means of exchanging knowledge across generations, knowledge that has been protected or regenerated by the Elders.

Nature can and should be drawn on in caring for Elders experiencing memory loss and/or diagnosed with dementia and could easily be integrated into recreational programming, particularly in facilities designed for small-group dementia care, with pods or hamlets. One such facility in the Interior of BC is in the planning stages of developing a hamlet – a unit that houses 14 residents – for First Nation Elders and has considered storytelling for youth, interior design, special menu planning, and Elders' luncheons as elements of culturally responsive care. Nature could be an element of all of these aspects of residential care, whether it be food that is drawn from the surrounding land or water, holding storytelling sessions with youth outdoors, or in combination with activities such as digging up the roots or growing tomatoes.

Nature-assisted therapy (Annerstedt and Wahrbourg 2011) has been implemented in dementia care and evaluated to a certain extent; the most common form to date has been horticulture therapy, with positive results being found in most of the dementia studies included in Annerstedt and Wahrbourg's (2011) systematic review. More recently, adventure therapy activities such as sailing trips have been developed for persons with dementia (see Chapter 3 and www.dementiaadventure.co.uk) and a pilot study of a walking-in-the-woods program found that 'there are potentially very significant physical, emotional and social benefits to people living with dementia visiting woods and being active out in nature' (Mapes 2011, p.3). Studies to date have not focused on particular socio-cultural groups such as First Nation Elders, however. Building on nature-assisted therapy in dementia care by introducing more culturally relevant programming such as berry picking, fishing, and gathering medicines as well as bringing the outdoors inside through activities such as canning salmon would be well received by First Nation Elders.

Concluding words

This chapter has attempted to provide insight into the integral role of nature for First Nation Elders concerned with preventing memory loss in later life and supporting one another as they respond to this new phenomenon called dementia. Dementia presents an opportunity to revive the practice of storytelling by Elders as it is thought to keep memory strong and can be a means by which Elders share knowledge with children; as such, storytelling can foster a greater understanding of one's interconnectedness with nature. Digging up the roots can lead to greater awareness of Secwepemc knowledge and traditions and a return to healthy lifestyles, which could potentially decrease risk factors for dementia.

The chapter ends with a quote from an Elder about the cycle of life and the interconnectedness of all those who live on the land, as it demonstrates the application of this belief system to practice in the form of the storyteller whose role is to remember and to remind others of the relativity of life:

> There is a cycle of life that I like when we sit in a circle; we should, we should get our own minds, hearts, and like plants and animals and the fish, and basically the world around us, you know that is what we are talking about is real, that we do eat

them and then, they do become part of us, they do heal us, and they do make up our home, and it's us who needs them, they don't necessar[ily] need us. We are the ones that need them, 'cause we can't do without them; they can do without us, but we can't do without them, and that's, that's the type of things that our people have said: we are the ones that need them to heal us, [it] takes away the mysteries of our life as passed on to us from them, more understanding and more, more respect for the things that help us continue our lives, even the air, you know, water, and that's, that comes through the storyteller, and remembering, remembering those things, everything was important, if it was created, then it was a relative, 'cause every part of it had a part of God in it when it was created.

(male, SC 4, Oct 2011)

Chapter 9

A Sense of Place

An Anthroposophic Approach

JUDITH JONES

Andy has put on his overcoat and is ready to go out to find his car. It is almost 9.00pm and we were hoping he would be on his way to bed. Andy has Lewy Body dementia and has not driven for years, but from time to time the memory of his beloved car wells up and he is determined to find it. The night nurse is arriving in a few minutes and it would be so good to have everyone settled for the night. But today there is no way of persuading Andy that his mission can wait until the morning. So off we go through the back door, complete with zimmer frame and up the path to the car park. There is already a chill in the air, but it is a clear night with a myriad of stars in the sky. Andy does not see any car but now thinks he might find his bicycle instead. We walk on until his legs begin to tire. Suddenly car and bicycle seem to be forgotten and he is willing to turn back. Coming down the path, our attention turns to the stars and we agree that it could be Jupiter that shines so brightly and that tomorrow it will probably be fine weather. By the time we get back through the door I am beginning to feel cold and Andy says his legs are aching. We are both ready for a cup of tea. It is almost half past nine but Andy gets happily into his pyjamas and I can leave in peace.

This is life in Simeon Care for the Elderly, a home for 17 older people of whom eight have a diagnosis of dementia. It is also home for others who work here and live on site, including young volunteers from different parts of the world. We have taken as our motto Jonathan Swift's words 'May you live all the days of your life'. Our aim is that everyone might embrace life fully and meaningfully. We value the importance of life sharing, having meals together, celebrating our comings and goings and, for some, sharing the roof over our heads.

We aspire to be a good nursing care home in the natural setting of an age-friendly community.

In whatever setting, living with and supporting those with dementia is a challenge to conventional encounters, testing our patience, openness and honesty. As carers we need to find new responses to unpredictable moods and reactions, to sense in the other the sometimes overwhelming power of colour, sound or scent, unbounded by notions of time and space. We need to discover what evokes memory or creates association of thoughts, what disturbs equilibrium or offers distraction. We are constantly exploring how to be with the other in the present moment.

The reality in which the person with dementia lives is often not comprehensible to our rational thinking. Living with those with dementia can give rise to existential questions about the meaning of life and relationships. The Austrian scientist and philosopher Rudolf Steiner (1861–1925) opened many views on the riddles of humanity. Anthroposophy, the collective word for his insights, encompasses a way of seeing a person not only as body and soul but as an eternal and evolving spirit. Anthroposophy considers that there is meaning and purpose in each phase and condition of our unfolding biographies.

Our health and wellbeing depends on a balanced relationship of body, soul and spirit which we see being thrown into imbalance in dementia. In Steiner's view, illness manifests itself primarily in body and soul while the spirit remains intact. It follows that for the person with dementia the spiritual need for recognition, respect and dignity does not change. Likewise, opportunities to experience beauty, rhythm and meaningful activity may contribute to letting spiritual integrity shine through the illness.

Steiner recognised a living reality of spirit in both the human being and the universe. He was described by Shepherd (1991) as a scientist of the invisible as he sought to investigate the working of phenomena not perceptible to the senses. Steiner pointed to the relationships we have not only with one another but also with all the life forces that surround us. He held the view that we are intimately linked with the natural world around and the starry universe beyond. The human body is made up of substances and processes that are found in nature, a key to the healing potential of plants and minerals. We are influenced by the same living forces and processes that unfold in the natural world, reflecting the rhythms of sun, moon and stars and manifesting through the seasonal variation of the year. As human beings we are not separate from the spirit at work in nature.

Camphill communities, known internationally for their work with children and adults with special needs, grew out of the inspiration of anthroposophy. Simeon Care for the Elderly, founded in the 1980s, was the first Camphill community specifically for older people. Simeon has been inspired by the ideal of 'life sharing' and has adopted and adapted much of its ethos from other Camphill settings. This means wanting to live in a healthy and wholesome way, using natural products, but also caring for the earth and respecting its resources. It also means attentiveness to the rhythms of nature from the daily rhythm to the seasonal course of the year.

Situated at the edge of Aberdeen, we are fortunate to be located on a beautiful estate with an open vista of green, encompassing flower beds and wild areas, a walled garden and orchard. There are beautiful trees with a path leading around the estate. The daughter of one of our residents writes:

> One of the attractions of Simeon in choosing a care home was the surrounding beautiful natural environment and the ease with which this environment could be entered, as all the living areas are on ground level. It is not simply a pretty garden, but an area of significant space, with ample shrubbery and a variety of large mature trees as well as the colourful displays created by garden flowers. In this environment the sky too becomes something bigger and of more significance.
>
> My mother Lily is 94 years old and was diagnosed with dementia eight years ago. Lily lives her life moment by moment, constantly trying to piece together fragments of memories that frequently slip out of reach; forever struggling to remember what she should be doing next. Does she have a job? Does she have family responsibilities? Is she in transit, going somewhere else? Where is she?
>
> Sometimes she calls me by name spontaneously; sometimes she has no memory beyond her own childhood and certainly cannot remember mine. Sometimes she can be content to sit with a cup of tea and chat, other times she is restless, distrustful,

angry and difficult. Especially in that mood, or to avert negative moods, the therapeutic value of nature is priceless.

I have been aware for some time now of the uplifting value of a simple walk immersed in nature, with Lily in a wheelchair and me at the rear, pushing. This has an undoubted calming effect, a sense of being grounded, perhaps a sense of belonging, and more than anything Lily wants to belong, but can't remember to what or to whom. Also nature very clearly illustrates time of day and time of year; it provides a focus for discussions in the present, when Lily's opinion has value. So many other everyday topics are out of her reach now, out of her comfort zone, and can expose her limitations.

These are my opinions however, so on recent walks I have questioned Lily to get an understanding of her view. Clarifying first of all that we were walking in the grounds of the place she is living, I asked how she felt about that. Her answer: 'Fortunate.' I told her I felt that nature lifted her spirits and asked if she agreed. She said that yes, she supposed that was the case, and so I asked why she thought nature had this effect. She replied that perhaps it was linked to childhood, something triggering the past.

For dementia sufferers, getting a perspective on life is challenging. Perhaps it's the simple fact that we all breathe better in nature, better air, and deeper, longer, slower breaths. Perhaps it's more positive inputs for all our senses; perhaps it's the pace of life in nature. Or perhaps it's something more fundamental to our being – I like the idea of that sense of belonging to something bigger, something non-judgemental.

To live closely with nature gives not only opportunities for daily walks or wheelchair rides but also opportunities to take part in meaningful activities that the surroundings offer. In spring there are flowers to pick and arrange. One of our residents has introduced the pressing of flowers to make cards and calendars. In summer there are berries to be picked and prepared for jam and juice making; in autumn help with the harvesting; and in winter feeding the birds and watching them on snowy days, or just sitting by the wood fire with logs that have come from trees that have over the years been felled on the estate.

We are fortunate to have regular deliveries of organic meat and vegetables, besides having some produce from our own gardens. We offer herb teas, made from fresh or dried herbs from our garden, as alternative options to coffee and tea. The majority of our residents are registered with the Camphill Medical Practice whose doctors prescribe natural medicines and care treatments in addition to allopathic medicine. Complementary treatments are supervised by qualified nurses. Andy was for a time given a weekly ginger compress over his kidneys to help to stimulate warmth and relaxation during a period of presenting challenging behaviour. The compress was prepared from freshly grated root ginger and its benefit was in helping him feel more at peace. As general care products, for those residents who would like them, we use rosemary bath milk in the washing water for wakening and lavender bath milk in the evening for relaxing.

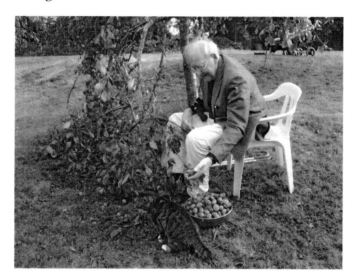

Figure 9.1 Andy harvesting plums

Another aspect of being connected to nature is finding ways to celebrate the seasonal course of the year with the highlights of religious festivals, in our case Christian festivals. At Easter we decorate our houses with spring flowers and branches hung with painted eggs. At the end of June we join our neighbours, a community for young adults with learning difficulties, around a bonfire in our grounds, enjoying watching the rising flames in this midsummer celebration. In autumn, we help with gathering the harvest from our walled garden, arranging a harvest table and sharing a meal together which is the produce from our own garden. During December, we make Advent wreaths, the scent of pine filling the house, and light candles to mark the way to Christmas. Finally, a few days before Christmas the tree arrives, waiting to be decorated, and there are preparations for Christmas dinner to be made.

Here in Scotland one of the favourite festivals is Burns Night towards the end of January. It is celebrated with the piping in and ceremonial stabbing of the haggis, followed by poetry and songs. The familiarity of these traditions and the nostalgia of the music have a particular appeal. The celebrations can be simple but the mood profound. For those with dementia who are losing their orientation in time, these familiar celebrations are meaningful landmarks in the year.

Amongst our residents who have dementia, several have been keen gardeners. Until two years ago Betty, who is now 97, was out gardening every day. This activity kept her going and seemed to slow the progress of her dementia. Whilst earlier she had planned and persevered with her flower beds, as her dementia set in and mobility simultaneously slowed down Betty would increasingly just potter in the garden. Wherever she would find herself, there would always be weeds to pick or dead growth to cut down. She was reluctant to use a walking stick but learned with the garden fork to appreciate a support. She eventually accepted a wheeled walker because its basket attachment provided an alternative wheelbarrow for transporting weeds to the compost heap. The physiotherapist who came to assess Betty's mobility said herself that there was no better activity than her continuing to work in the garden. When walking and bending down became too risky we found another occupation, which was sawing wood. A sawhorse and small branches were set up outside the window so we were able to keep an eye on her. She ingeniously used her zimmer frame to stack the wood. The last phase of Betty's garden activity was a self-created task – gathering fir cones for kindling for the fire. She ingeniously managed to pick them up with her 'helping hand' reaching aid and put them into the basket of her walker. Many fires have been lit with the help of Betty's fir cones.

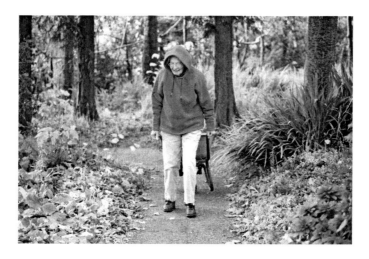

Figure 9.2 Betty with her wheelbarrow off to the wood pile

Another resident, Catherine, tells elaborate and fascinating stories of things she has done in her full and active life. In these tales she often uses nature imagery, and listening behind her words can give a sense of how she is metaphorically describing what is going on inside herself. She will tell of climbing mountains or crossing rivers, as if she herself is journeying into new and unfamiliar territories. Sometimes Catherine experiences a sense of being guided and supported – 'Someone took my hand when I crossed the river.' On another occasion when Catherine was very despondent she said, 'I got stuck in the mud and couldn't get out.' Catherine's brother has written of the inner change he has observed occurring through her dementia. She had been strongly independent and assertive, but in her growing dependency a new softness began to show itself. He writes:

> When some years ago the dementia was beginning I could observe some changes of behaviour and character. Instead of becoming cross Catherine showed a side of her character which was rather unknown before. She became mild and friendly. I could observe that Catherine's severity and sharpness changed into friendliness, mildness and softness. Maybe those who care for Catherine now mainly experience the many difficulties. But the essence of her character is what became obvious at the

onset of her dementia, this mildness and devotion which she had previously hidden.

Catherine's mother had been a gardener and she had grown up in a home with a large garden. Although training as a physiotherapist, Catherine herself had spent most of her working life as a gardener. Her niece adds some thoughts about her connection to nature. She writes:

> Catherine's contact with plants and trees is very direct. I notice this each time we walk around Simeon's grounds and stop here and there so that my aunt can admire the beauty of a rose opening its petals and smell its fragrance. Catherine welcomes the trees we pass. She loves to compare the trees we look at with those I mention from our home surroundings and which she can remember from her childhood. It feels good for her to talk about the old chestnut trees in front of her parents' house and how they unfolded their finger-like leaves and opened their white blossoms when her birthday came in May.
>
> To live with nature so nearby seems to offer Catherine a sense of wellbeing and consolation. I dare say that it has a relaxing and reassuring effect on her as her dementia is marked by a fear of loss, of losing her memory and the beloved people of her childhood. She desperately needs contacts that can restore her feeling of security.
>
> Her deep appreciation of nature is depicted in stories she tells again and again. One story she has created is now well known to all in Simeon. The story goes that Catherine had climbed up Lochnagar, a high peak in the nearby Scottish highlands. After reaching the summit there was a sudden snowstorm and Catherine was soon lost, frozen and exhausted. Then she saw children coming towards her, some even with crutches, and they took her under her arms and led her step by step down the mountain slope. The story has a number of variations but usually ends with finding a warm water bottle in her bed when she finally arrived home safely.
>
> I shall never forget my aunt's bright eyes when on my first visit to her in Simeon we were able to visit a nearby Camphill community where Catherine had earlier in her life worked as a

gardener. Despite her disorientation Catherine led me straight to a place at the edge of the garden, pointed to a nearly illegible plaque set in the old stone wall and asked me to read the following lines:

A kiss of the sun for pardon
The song of the bird for mirth
You're nearer God's heart in a garden
Than anywhere else on earth.

Catherine helped me to make out the weathered letters as she knew the poem by heart and was in tears as if delivering her own message. I would go as far as to say that my aunt's dementia has allowed her to express her subconscious feelings as if sheltering the fragile and tender part of her that she had always found difficult to express.

Maisy, a former resident, had supported her husband with his market garden besides other outlets for sharing her many artistic and musical gifts. We experienced her creativity when she first came to Simeon and would gather and arrange countless objects of natural beauty. What was touching to experience was that as her dementia developed the profusion of items she gathered diminished. Two of Maisy's daughters describe this process:

All through her life Maisy collected stones, cones, feathers, pressed leaves and flowers with a view, most of the time, to find something useful 'to do' with them, such as creating painted stones, pressed flower cards or decorated cones for Christmas. She had a keen eye for such things and an imagination to visualise what she could do with half a walnut shell or a sprig of honesty seed cases.

Throughout her illness she still collected and received great peace and contentment from a leisurely stroll along the canal in Edinburgh where she lived, or later in the gardens at Simeon. However, one could observe a change in her collecting as her illness progressed. She once remarked that colours had become brighter and more luminous when she looked at them and that around many objects, flowers or lights she saw a rainbow-coloured halo.

In Edinburgh, a year or so before she made her home in Simeon, the loss of inhibitions would find her opening a garden gate along her street in order to pick a particular flower which caught her attention! Or to pause while in the middle of a cycle way to stare into a clover patch and search for a four-leaf clover, which she invariably found and then offered to a complete stranger with a smiling comment, 'Do you want to get lucky?'

From all her forays into nature, whether a country walk with the family, or a wander around an abandoned derelict corner of the city, she would return with bunches of flowers, handfuls of coloured leaves or budding twigs. There was a time when in her flat every available surface was occupied with vases of flowers, twigs or seed-heads, often 15 or more in all different shapes and sizes of vase. Each day she would take them out and refill the vases, cut off dead flower heads, wilted leaves, etc., and rearrange them in different combinations of colour or structure and then replace them all around the house.

When first arriving in Simeon Maisy found her greatest pleasure in wandering the grounds, returning with bunches of leaves and flowers that initially she would arrange artistically in vases, but as time went on that task failed her. However, she still picked and gathered. Now she would often return with a strange bunch of objects which had caught her eye: a leaf with a bite out of it, a browned seed-head from a docken plant, a minute blue-tinged feather. As she stiffened and slowed up, and was latterly wheeled in a chair, she was almost silent until she spied something in a group of grasses, amongst the weeds of a compost heap, or at the edge of the path. We would be directed to either pick or gather it up. We would often have to be directed repeatedly until we found the exact object which had caught her eye. It might just be a small shrivelled-up red leaf. She still saw the beauty in the object which we recognised as something that was dying, ugly or past its best.

As other skills left her, like her words, ability to move and comprehension of daily life, she still retained a powerful and amazing sense of colour and form in nature. A pebble along a gravel path might catch her eye, but only after one stopped, picked it up and looked closely at it did one observe the small quartz corner that had glinted at her in the sun.

Alzheimer's seemed to pare away so much of Maisy over the years, but underneath it all the essence of her remained true: her keen eye for colour and form and her love of nature, most especially the plant world, and the peace it always brought her when she could spend time whatever the weather, in a white hat and red coat, just being in its embrace.

Maisy had a very sunny side to her nature and had a favourite song she would sing and try to teach to others: 'It is summer, it is summer, how beautiful it looks, there's sunshine on the old grey hills and sunshine on the brooks...' She would sing it winter and summer alike. Somehow it seemed to express who she was. When after her funeral service in our hall the coffin was driven away, those gathered to make their farewell spontaneously broke into this summer song.

Death is a part of life. We talk about wanting a good death surrounded by our loved ones and in our familiar setting. Many of our families have expressed the meaningfulness of the last days or weeks of accompanying a relative. As the wife of one of our former residents wrote:

> I wish to thank you, from the bottom of my heart, for your loving care and kindness towards John during his illness and death, and for your care for me! I will always remember this period of my life as a very special time, full of beauty, dignity and love. It was like a magical time, where all fell into place in 'unthought-of' ways – when heaven and earth touched each other.

For those residents and families who wish it, we let the open coffin remain in the resident's room for up to three days after death, surrounded by flowers and candlelight. This old tradition of a 'wake' is an opportunity for the other residents, carers, family and friends to pay their last respects and, if they wish, sit for a while by the coffin. It is a time to offer comfort and support to one another and for those remaining in the house to experience the peace and gentleness that can accompany the departing. Many funerals take place in our hall and can be rich celebrations of life. After the funeral we often gather with the family to share our memories of the person who has died.

Whilst situated in natural surroundings, we also have the benefit of modern technology in our home, with all manner of profiling beds, hoists and electric chairs which facilitate our care work. Yet equipment also challenges us to develop our sensitivity, particularly with residents with dementia who, despite explanation, cannot grasp what may be happening to them. Betty goes through phases when she is fearful of any movement. On occasions the stand aid is needed to assist Betty. It appears to her as a monster that immediately instils fear. Faced with extreme sensitivities the quality of touch becomes of great importance. Sometimes we are able to restore her sense of security through gentle touch, lightly massaging her hands or feet.

The sense of separation which the word dementia implies leads to anxiety, insecurity, fear and confusion, and ultimately to a mistrust of the world around and a weakening of personal identity. Betty once had a strong grip on life and in her slowly developing dementia has often been able to express her sense of losing herself. Betty is now receiving help through the Camphill Medical Practice with sessions of movement therapy. Her therapist explains:

> Movement is a natural process of transformation that can help in finding oneself and one's connections. The human voice, touch and warmth, a calm presence and peaceful movements can go a long way towards providing possibilities for relieving anxiety, offering reassurance and providing the ground for trust to develop, also a chance to re-identify with aspects of herself. I try to provide for Betty an experience of feeling whole again. To begin the session I want to give a sense of being present, of not being hurried, offering an unthreatening ambience. I hold Betty's hands with a warm tender touch, stroke arms and gently massage hands and feet. These gestures can help to bring an awareness of her own hands and feet and help build some identity with her body, offering a sense of security. Using oils with natural scents, for example lavender, creates not only a calm soothing atmosphere but can trigger pleasant memories of childhood or gardens. A conversation may start: 'Do you like the scent? Can you recognise the smell?' Betty says, 'My mother used to grow lavender in her garden.' With these preliminary gestures I attempt to move on and engage more. I suggest to Betty to try using hands and feet again now they are nice and warm.

After taking time to feel the arms of the chair and making good contact with her feet on the ground it is possible to take a few steps around the room, arm in arm together. Gentle encouraging to stand and to sit and to experience the feet one in front of the other may offer Betty an increasing experience of herself. The next stage of introducing any other movements is possible only if the preparatory steps have been made. These attempts are not about getting from A to B. They are a therapeutic attempt to create the setting for a natural movement process to take place, hopefully benefiting Betty by having an experience of 'wholeness' again.

An irony of our time is that while computer technology is enabling us to store more information and gain access to ever more knowledge, the growing phenomenon of dementia is taking away the very power of memory and ability to process information. Instead of mastery we are faced with helplessness and despair. Neither for the person with dementia nor his carer are there blueprints for how to cope, but trials to be lived through. Yet we may sometimes be aware that dementia is challenging us in a particular way to discover new dimensions of relationship. A daughter of Maisy made the remark during the last weeks of her mother's life that in her passive state she had been able to meet her mother in a quite new way.

I always marvel at how our young volunteer carers are drawn towards two highly dependent residents, both with Down's syndrome in their last stage of dementia. When asked to describe the experience of caring for them, one young person said:

It is a challenge to know them at first when they cannot say anything, but now I know them I can read how they feel in their eyes, sometimes through a smile or expression of pain. They are so open, so easy to read, so our communication is very open. It is both giving and receiving. I sense something very pure.

Rudolf Steiner gave a particular view on the blessings of old age. He spoke about the possibility of reliving and processing one's biography even in a state of disorientation. He also recognised that as older people's bodies grow frailer their spirituality becomes more freely available for others. Steiner was once asked why an old lady who was both paralysed and unconscious should still be alive. She needed intensive care, and it was suggested to him that it might be more humane to allow her to die. Steiner said, 'No, every day, every hour she lives on earth is not only a boon for her but is of meaning for the whole of humanity' (Gaumnitz 2009).

Living with those with dementia brings its trials, its joys and sorrows, its disappointments and failings. It challenges us to reflect on ourselves and our attitudes and responses. It brings also the challenge to look at life differently and to consider how we are affected by the world around us. Through all the stages and phases of confusion, disorientation and loss of self-awareness, we can only try to uphold dignity and integrity in the face of situations which can become stressful to those with dementia and those around them. In Simeon we recognise that one positive way of alleviating stress is by maintaining what is natural and familiar. The little things in life grow in importance – the daily greetings, the flowers on the table or a cup of tea together. The simplest things can bring the most joy – opportunities to peel vegetables, to look out at the changing weather or go for walks in the garden. These are opportunities life gives us to restore the familiar, to share experience and to allow the healing and harmonising spirit in nature to work. Nature has the power to lift our spirits. In its presence and solace it is no wonder that the mother principle in nature has been long recognised. In the words of Catherine's niece:

> Nature has no boundaries. In its global and generous way it welcomes everyone, never judging anyone's behaviour, like a mother waiting for her child to come home after a long, long journey.

Chapter 10

Nature in the Lives of an Urban Population with Dementia in North East England

KAREN FRANKS AND KATE ANDREWS

Introduction

Our interest in exploring our clients' relationship with nature was sparked by reading about others' experiences in Gilliard and Marshall's first book on nature and dementia (2011). It was good to see a subject which we had been discussing appear in such an accessible and varied book. We felt, however, that it did not really reflect many of the experiences of the natural world that were talked about by the people with dementia we work with. We work in Gateshead in the North East of England. Its population is predominantly white British, mainly urban and working class. Mining and manufacturing were the main employers of the generation, industries that have since disappeared or declined significantly. Historically the housing was rows of brick terraces of small houses with tiny yards behind them or flats with limited, if any, outside space.

Those we work with have talked to us in the past about allotments and pigeon lofts, municipal parks and rare trips to the seaside. Given this, we were curious as to how our clients with dementia connected to the natural world then, and whether there was a sense of relationship with it now. We wanted to try to capture these experiences. We hoped that they could help in our understanding and guide appropriate provision for more people with dementia in the future.

There is much literature available regarding the importance of being able to go outdoors for people with dementia (Pollock and Marshall 2012). However, a significant issue in many care settings is residents' limited experiences of being outside (see Care Commission and Mental Welfare Commission 2009, for example). In our experience, while the care homes provide outside spaces, often employing much thought and consideration in the garden setting, residents' time in this space is often limited. Anecdotally this would appear to be either reduced staffing levels or anxieties regarding residents' safety (for example, the risk of falls) which inhibits these activities.

We approached two local residences for people with dementia whose managers and residents were willing to work with us. The first was a Promoting Independence Centre specifically for people with dementia run by Gateshead Council. It has 23 beds and provides planned and emergency respite services, assessment beds and some day services. It has a central garden that is well used. A recent addition has been their chickens, which have been extremely popular with residents and visitors. Such has been their popularity that they have been featured in local and national newspapers in recent months. The second was a privately run home with 66 beds, providing 24-hour care for people with dementia in both residential and nursing settings. It has some outside space, which is not often used, but it does run regular trips out and encourages residents to go out with family, friends and staff when possible.

Into these two different settings we took a number of items from our own gardens and surrounding areas to generate discussion. We took home-grown vegetables (many with soil attached), herbs, compost, grass, hay, flowers and autumn leaves and set up a 'nature table'. In the first setting, residents were invited to visit the table and talk about their thoughts. In the second, we found taking two small tables to individuals and small groups of residents worked better as they were less mobile. We asked people about their experiences of nature currently as well as in the past and recorded their responses on portable recorders.

We analysed the responses using Interpretative Phenomenological Analysis (IPA). According to Smith and Osborn (2003) the main aim of IPA is to explore in detail how participants make sense of their personal and social world. The approach is from a phenomenological perspective and therefore it involves a detailed exploration of the participant's experience with the focus being the individual's account or perception of the phenomena. The objective of IPA is the account given by the participant, as opposed to an objective statement of the event. Similar to other qualitative methodologies, the role of the researcher is central to the process, and IPA emphasises that research is a dynamic process with an active role for the researcher. Given that the objective of the research is to understand and gain an 'insider perspective' (Conrad 1987), the preconceptions of the researcher might restrict this. Smith and Osborn suggested that these ideas are required to make sense of the participant's world through an interpretative process.

Emergent themes

Source of food

Participants were asked about whether they had access to outside space when younger. Despite living in urban areas, many of the participants recalled the homes having allotments or backyards which had been adapted for use as vegetable plots:

> 'Dad grew vegetables for the whole family and used to give to neighbours and to old people.'

> 'I remember Dad growing them [pointing to potatoes]...used to think can't eat them, too small.'

One lady recalled that having a vegetable plot made 'everyone the same', suggesting that the vegetable plots gave a sense of community and equality.

Several of our participants spoke of the vegetables providing not only a source of food, but also a sense of pride:

> 'My husband grew leeks for the shows. They were very good.'

Leisure time

A prominent theme when speaking with the participants was the sense that being outside was important to leisure time. For many of the participants the limited individual space meant that they used the local parks, as travelling outside the local area was expensive:

'Didn't get into the countryside as [I] lived on the high street… couldn't afford to get to the countryside.'

'I was bred and born on the Teams so I used to go to the park a lot, it was at the top of the street, it was nice.'

'I lived on the high street, we didn't have gardens…it was busy.'

'We used to go [to] the "Hikey" park.'

Recall of the local park appeared to evoke positive memories:

'When I was young used to go to Saltwell Park and bowl with eggs in the summertime. The flowers always bloomed in the summer. It's one of the best…something for everyone.'

'It was nice to go to Saltwell Park…it was a canny walk.'

'I grew up with the Park. I chased the girls there.'

One lady recalled her late husband having an allotment and spoke of how she had enjoyed her time in that space:

'I used to sit in a deckchair and relax…only time I got until the kids grew up.'

However, the parks were not always available for everyone, and therefore people spoke of other places they went to:

'Used to go up near the railway line as there were swans there.'

'I love the fresh air…I used to walk for miles with the dog.'

'Used to take the bairns down to the cemetery for a walk.'

Balance

Many of our participants or their families worked in an industrial setting, including brick factories, steel mills and coal mines. Their narrative suggested that being outside engaged in some activity provided some sense of contrast to their daily activities:

'My father was a miner and he had a mass of wallflowers. I think that was what made him have lots of wallflowers.'

'My husband was a good grower when he wasn't down the pits.'

A lady recalled her late husband's racing pigeons:

> 'He enjoyed them. I used to say to him that you would rather [have] the pigeons than me [laughing]. I suppose he needed them as he was down the pit a lot.'

Reminiscence

Seeing the prompts appeared to evoke memories of family for many participants:

> 'My parents, my garden and all my home and that…it all comes back.'

> 'I see my bungalow with snowdrops and the trees.'

Loss

A sense of loss was apparent in many of the narratives when asked about their experiences now of being outside. Many spoke about deficits within their own health that might prevent them getting outside:

> 'Don't get out and about…I have no legs.'

Or not having someone to take them out:

> 'My family works and my husband is dead…don't get out now.'

Or simply that they just don't go:

> 'I miss being outside.'

Discussion

Our findings put into context nature in the lives of a population who grew up in a very urbanised setting. Throughout their lives they sought out ways to connect with the natural world. They used nature as a way to bring balance to their lives and their emotional state. For example, our sample reminisced of growing flowers in the garden, of walking and socialising in the parks. Growing vegetables provided them not only with a source of nutrients, but also a sense of equality and pride in their achievements. Our impression from their accounts suggests that an opportunity was never wasted to utilise and value any available outside space, whether for flowers or vegetables.

Our experience of our sample is that they had become disconnected from this relationship with nature. As practitioners, we considered what effects this lack of contact with the natural world might have. We wonder whether this may add further to the loss of sense of purpose that appears to be experienced by many with dementia. Could it be engendering a feeling of being constantly at work and deprived of leisure? Could this then be perceived as a loss of liberty or even punishment? These findings add to our sense that those with dementia in a care setting are often deprived of community and shared experiences.

A significant question from our research is simply: 'Why do people in care settings have apparently little or no access to the natural world?' We have considered a number of factors that might explain this phenomenon. For example, has the 'care system' truly considered the benefits of this to their population, or is it that 'care' only happens within four walls? Lack of awareness, lack of training for activity coordinators and lack of recognition of need all seem to be factors.

Recommendations

The themes that come out of our sample demonstrate the purposefulness and functionality of the relationship with nature and how it is an integral part of an individual's sense of identity.

From our small sample it appears to us that what is important is the meaning that people give to their experiences, not necessarily the activities that they do. It would seem appropriate to consider re-creating these environments – outside spaces looking like a park, and vegetable plots and growing vegetables. Contact with nature is not only pleasurable, but it can be a source of pride, liberty and leisure, and can give a sense of doing something purposeful.

Conclusion

Unfortunately, moving into a 24-hour care setting often means isolation away from an individual's normal community and from the natural world. Care providers need to recognise the importance of the connection with nature. The recent architecture of care settings seems to reject this need in favour of fitting in a few more beds. Sometimes roof gardens are seen as a viable alternative but are then poorly accessible and rarely used. From our research, we suggest that a garden or space that resembles a park might be beneficial. Nature within the home is not happening – there are plastic plants and the outside world is rarely brought in except on the coats of visitors. With time, residents may become more disconnected from nature, especially as their physical health declines and their dementia worsens. Our study highlights that this connection with nature is as important to an urban population as to a rural one, although at times the meanings may be different.

We feel that these findings only serve to highlight the fact that the care of people with dementia often does not respect or identify people's relationships – with others, with their community and with the world. There is a pervasive lack of awareness of how connected we are to everything and everyone.

Chapter 11

Memories of an Urban Childhood with a Nearby Wood

JAMES MCKILLOP, MBE

I was born in a tenement in a (then) small town, close to a wood, and over the boundary wall was a field.

It was a room and kitchen and, with six of us siblings, we were encouraged to play outside. Luckily, in those days, the weather was fine and even hot. I remember walking with the Co-operative pipe band on the annual Gala Day out and my gutties got stuck in the melted tar on the road, and I, and others, ended up in bare feet. Looking back, I wonder how my mother ever got our feet clean again. I suppose she used household goods such as butter, but that was still on ration. We would end up at a park and drink milk in white enamel tin cups from large urns. The Co-op provided all sorts of buns, the cream ones being my favourite. In those days it was a real treat getting a bun. However, I digress.

The dyke, which barred us from the field, was about six feet tall. As we grew up and our muscles developed, we used toe holds to climb up and over. The top was quite broad and you could comfortably sit and rest after your exertions. A whole new world was opened to us. Green, green grass and a pond full of wildlife. I remember catching tadpoles and getting a jam jar (which was later exchanged to gain admission to the pictures, a common custom back then) to take them home. When they turned into frogs, they drowned. We did not realise that they needed air to breathe. Due to our ignorance, we inadvertently killed them. I also remember prying under rocks and disturbing all sorts of coloured newts. They outshone the clothes we wore, as fabrics were scarce after the war. We used to take them to the roof of the wash house (you were allocated a day to do your washing in the big boiler) and race them. To my shame, I do not recall if we returned them to the wild.

There were also numerous varieties of wild flowers and we always took some home as a peace offering, as we were invariably covered in mud. My favourite was a bunch of yellow dandelions, which looked very pretty. I know they are regarded as a weed, but gather them and really examine. They rival the best carnations in looks and colour. It was marvellous when they turned to seed. We blew them to tell the time, and they became known as dandelion clocks. But I think our stomachs told us much better when it was time to eat. There was mint growing wild and we would gather the leaves for our mother to make with dinner.

The wood was a short walk away and I found I could skim to the top of a tree quite easily and view the surrounding area, pretending I was in a plane. I will never know how I never fell off. The trees were a guide to the seasons. Stark and naked during the winter and budding green as spring advanced. The autumn was my favourite, as when the leaves turned golden it was time for chestnuts. Even to this day, at age 72, I still gather a chestnut or two and carry them in my pocket until the next autumn. As I sit here, I currently have four in my pocket. Toys were scarce, not just due to unavailability, but no one had money to buy them. We were too busy scraping a living. So we made our own fun. I used fallen branches to make a bow and arrows. I found greater accuracy if I tied a nail to the tip of the arrow. Luckily I never aimed at a person, just wood. What would H&S make of it these days? Apart from providing me with bows and arrows, the woods produced branches to be used as swords – well used after a matinee at the local flea pit, when we saw swashbuckling musketeers on the silver screen.

You could dine at the edge of the woods. I could always find raspberries, wild strawberries, red berries, blackcurrants and gooseberries to keep me going until I got home.

While I now hate snow, in case I fall, I absolutely loved it as a child. From building snowmen to topless forts, which we guarded with fearless zeal, to slides, which I hope nobody ever slipped on. I particularly remember 1947. The men in the block carved tunnels to gain access to the street. As I slithered along, the top of the snow was way over my child-size head. I now shudder to think it might have caved in and smothered me or others. If I remember correctly, that was also the year the moon was a blue colour, a source of wonderment to many.

No TV or computer games in those days but we had nature at our fingertips.

There was no National Health Service in those days, so we became our own doctors. Small cuts and grazes were treated with leaves. I particularly remember that when stung with stinging nettles (as opposed to stings from something like thistles) we would tear off a docken leaf and rub it on the affected part.

So with snowballs in winter, nature provided me with plenty of free toys, as money was scarce.

Chapter 12

Dementia and Landscapes

Cultural Attitudes Towards Nature

JOAN DOMICELJ

Preamble

While the natural world nourishes us as a species in universal ways, individual communities learn to respond to their particular environments in ways that are distinct and become embedded over time. So, our cultures, in language, thought and customs, are as diverse as the physical habitats to which we have adapted.

The familiar offers comfort; displacement from usual surroundings is a challenge. The presence of earth, sky and life around us may be constant but their fluctuating characteristics are not. Migrants experience disorientation when moved out of their normal surroundings; people with dementia even more poignantly. Maybe we can provide them with something of the familiar outdoors in sight, sound, smell, touch and habitual tasks.

Across the Asia Pacific region, people interact with nature in diverse ways. The differences are most marked within traditional cultures that have evolved over centuries. Later in this chapter we look at three examples of landscapes on UNESCO's World Heritage List. They are places of outstanding universal value that have acquired specific cultural meanings for their inhabitants. Further, within multicultural Australia, two migrant communities – the Macedonian and the Vietnamese – have been shown to adopt notably different attitudes towards national parks. These attitudes may give us a clue as to what, outdoors, may be most satisfying to those communities in old age. The process of caring for people with dementia may be enhanced by an understanding of their active lives in previous very different settings.

I have that strange feeling, a strange feeling,
Of a floating, shifting stream of saltwater…
Look!
I'm frightened,
I haven't been here before!

(Song poem of Andrew, an Aboriginal man from
the Coorong, as he moves between familiar
freshwater and alien saltwater countries)

The outdoors

'Nature deficit disorder describes the human costs of alienation from nature,' wrote Richard Louv in 2005. A 2012 study shows that most English children no longer walk to school, run errands or roam the neighbourhood. They are held indoors by electronics and 'well-meaning protective house arrest'. Sedentary life diminishes their physical and social skills, health, independence and ability to assess and cope with risk. Adults, and especially those with dementia, often experience similar restraints, with similar unhappy consequences.

The vital link between human health, both mental and physical, and access to nature is now accepted. The outdoor world offers certain forms of stimulus or reassurance to us all, in either known or newly discovered places. The need for dementia patients to spend time outside is recognised, but in what setting?

Particular comfort comes from known surroundings and the familiarity of sensations, activities and thoughts that accompany them. Their absence is what has frightened Andrew, in his song poem above. Each person's sense of place is based on culture and geography. It differs across communities and among individuals. It is drawn from where and how we have lived before, and with whom. It implants a sense of identity that is likely to continue throughout life. Earliest memories remain embedded, frequently into dementia.

An Israeli friend said that the perfume of figs or orange blossom brings tears to her eyes; for a Hungarian it was the taste of dill; for another it was soft, springy surfaces to walk on – not paving; another loved a painted landscape that I thought too dark – 'Remember, I come from Buffalo winters,' she said. All I had to do for an immediate response was to ask.

The universal

Already in the third century BC, the love of gardens could be strong. Greek naturalist and philosopher Theophrastus grew and classified 450 plants that were useful as food or medicine – and just a few garland flowers for their beauty. He so loved his garden that he left it to his slaves, who were to be freed on condition that they maintained it.

On our spaceship earth, land, sea and sky make up our habitat. We walk on the ground. We stand, sit and lie on it. The land is stable beneath our feet. It is where we live, work, sleep and play. It sustains and, sometimes, challenges us. The sea can be the same for those who live and work on it, though more tremulous.

So much for the land and sea. Now for the sky. With heads in the air, we share the sky above – radiant, clouded or sprinkled with stars. We breathe the air and wonder at the infinity of space. Here we think, question, invent, create and dream. As it was for our forefathers, our inspiration, stories and hopes are shaped by all that surrounds us.

The desert dweller may squint at the straight and distant horizon, with a hot wind on his face; for alpine people, the edges of sight may be rugged and the air bitterly cold. Yet, in both these different worlds, feet remain firm on the ground and heads are lifted towards the sky – universal.

The specific

A respected Indian social scientist and friend, Moonis Raza, wrote:

> Cultural identity is the fragrance of the earth, the myths we live on and legends that sustain us, the ballads that we sing and our concepts of heaven and hell.

We use our five senses to recognise the landscapes where we belong and the familiar activities there. Our minds hold our own memories, as well as stories told by our nurturing culture. Beyond the known lie other places, waiting to expand our understanding of a world that is as culturally rich in the diversity of its languages and songs as it is biologically rich in its landscapes. In caring for people with dementia we will concentrate on the known – and, it is hoped, those aspects that have been loved.

Australia still retains the oldest continuous cultures in the world. This is how Paddy Fordham Wainburranga, a Rembarrnga man, spoke of his country in Arnhem Land and its custodial law of singing:

> All the trees and the birds are your relations. There are different kinds of birds here. They can't talk to you straight up. You've got to sing out to them so they can know you…that's why I talked to the birds this morning, and all the birds were happy and sang out.

Imagine if he, as an old man with dementia, were to be confined to a place without those birds or trees. It would take his family away.

It should be remembered that close associations with landscapes are not always positive. It is customary in Australia for Aboriginal elders to welcome people to their traditional country at the opening of significant events. I remember a moving moment at the launch of an exhibition. The traditional owner explained, with obvious discomfort, that on this occasion he could only acknowledge the visitors and wish them well. This was bad country that should never have been developed – and so he could not welcome us to it. Caution is important. The known may be painful – we come once again to the importance of asking.

A single landscape may also inspire conflicting responses. I met Masuo Ikeda, eminent Japanese artist, writer and potter, in 1995 at a symposium on Mount Fuji. He shocked the huge local audience by shouting, 'I hate Mount Fuji!' What he hated was its slick adoption as a symbol of both nationalism and commercialism. On the other hand, he felt such a profound love for the place that he had created a beautiful painted ceramic series called '100 views of Mount Fuji', as seen from its graceful 'backside'. It is a place so embedded in his identity that it is likely to remain significant for him into old age. He also explained the celebratory importance of the sense of touch:

> Ceramic art is an effort to restore clay back to stone… After I began pottery work, my home-coming to Japan began.

Intense adult exposure to exceptional landscapes may remain seared in the mind in old age, as well as the familiar places of childhood. At the outbreak of the Second World War, a young German geologist called Henno Martin, his colleague (both of whom wanted none of it) and their dog fled into the harsh Namib Desert in Namibia and hid there for two and a half years. They somehow survived, hoarding remnant water, hunting elusive prey and pondering profound questions of human existence. Martin wrote about it decades later:

> The magic of the desert is hard to define. Why does the sight of a landscape of empty sand, rocks, slab and rubble stir the spirits more than a view of lush green fields and woods?... Perhaps... because the mind of the beholder is presented with a mirage of unlimited freedom.

At least two knowledge systems affect human relations with the land – the scientific and the traditional. Great wisdom can be achieved when their insights and expertise are shared – and comfort granted when respect is shown to both.

Here is an example. In Ghana, savanna ecosystems had suffered from slash-and-burn farming practices over many, many years. In 1992, an international team was appointed to advise on re-afforesting the severely damaged land. Scientists arrived to find that the only patches of indigenous vegetation that had survived for them to study were small sacred groves, fiercely protected by animist priests for ritual and religious practices. The scientists had to earn the trust of the priests by showing a proper respect for their beliefs and customs before controlled access was allowed and knowledge could be exchanged between science and tradition. This was to the great benefit of the country, through a mutually supported program of revegetation. The place remained the same, but the stories and meanings were different, and custodianship of the land was improved through sharing.

World heritage

UNESCO's World Heritage Convention (1972) celebrates and protects extraordinary cultural and natural places around the world that are found to be of 'outstanding universal value' and, so, are inscribed on the World Heritage List. Over recent years, its Committee has considered the subtleties of places such as cultural landscapes, where natural attributes are infused with meaning by associated cultural ties. Communities differ profoundly in how they perceive, and are attached to, landscapes. So, in seeking the universal, the Committee now takes into account the specifics of cultural associations.

Here are three examples of World Heritage properties in the Asia Pacific region. In 1995, the Japanese Historic Villages of Shirakawa-go and Gokayama were inscribed on the World Heritage List, followed, in 2000, by the Australian Greater Blue Mountains Area and, in 2010, by the Historic Villages of South Eastern Korea: Hahoe and Yangdong. All were recognised as places of 'outstanding universal value'.

In each place, particular cultural practices have evolved over long periods of time, in response to the specifics of the physical environment. The communities belonging there are surrounded by familiar sights and sounds and have grown used to specific ways of thinking and behaving.

The Historic Villages of Shirakawa-go and Gokayama

The village of Ogimachi is one of the 'Historic Villages of Shirakawa-go and Gokayama – Traditional Houses in the Gassho Style'. It lies along a river bank in an isolated, mountainous region of Japan that was, for 12 centuries, the focus for ascetic religious mountain worship. Its guardian deity is housed in a Shinto shrine at the base of the mountain, surrounded by a cedar grove and abutted by rice fields.

The village subsists on cultivating mulberry trees and rearing silkworms. Its steeply pitched Gassho thatched roofs enclose the silkworm beds and stored mulberry leaves. The region relies on co-operation among households for communal activities, such as re-thatching roofs and fire-fighting, and, despite various economic upheavals, traditional life continues to suit its environment and circumstances.

So what would a person with dementia, if displaced from this village, most warm to in a new setting? There are hints: perhaps the sight and perfume of mulberries or cedars, the sound of flowing water, the touch of straw or silk, the taste of rice – even a distant mountain and shrine – and, perhaps most importantly, the chance to join in indoor and outdoor tasks, in community with others.

The Greater Blue Mountains Area

I myself live in the Greater Blue Mountains Area of Australia, in a raft-like house hovering at the escarpment's edge. Over a million hectares of sandstone plateaux with deeply incised valleys were World Heritage listed in 2000, principally for their rich eucalypt-related biodiversity and protective habitats for endangered species. However, as a wild landscape, it has cultural values too. It is cherished by Aboriginal people from six language groups and by other poets and artists, bushwalkers and rangers, bird-watchers and people abseiling off cliffs.

I wrote a dedication once:

> Mt Korrowal ripples across the horizon, sharp-edged or shrouded in mists, crossed by shrieking cockatoos and hidden Yowies. The valley floor, 300 metres below, is blue-grey with eucalypts and filled with the sounds of spilling water and birds – when on fire it roars, as dangerous as the sea. Today is chock-a-block with avian shouts and sudden flashes – kookaburra, currawong and blue-red rosellas a metre from my face. Below, the hum of bellbirds and other small creatures. Sploshes of water and deep cascade rumbles. Twigs, seedpods, lizards and insects clicking and rustling their scratchy bush lyrics. Glorious.

The scent of eucalypt, the wild weather, scratchy bark scatters and the bird sounds affect us all. In old age, we may well rely on them for comfort.

The Historic Villages of South Eastern Korea: Hahoe and Yangdong

In 2010, the 'Historic Villages of South Eastern Korea: Hahoe and Yangdong' were inscribed on the World Heritage List. They are said to epitomise the Confucian principles of the Joseon Dynasty (1392–1910) – harmoniously composed within the landscape and with a visible social structure:

> If there are no mountains and streams, emotions cannot be good and people will be coarse. If mountains and rivers are engaged

from afar, people will harbour ambition, but if they are engaged
closely people's minds will be pure and their spirits joyful.

> (*Primer for Choosing Settlements*,
> Yi Jung-hwan, 1690–1756)

Cooking smoke rises straight above each house…
It screens the glare of the autumn glow.

> (*16 Beautiful Sceneries in Hahoe*,
> poems by Ryu Won-ji, 1598–1674)

I visited the clan villages in 2008 in that 'glare of the autumn glow'
– shimmering red, gold, citrus foliage on mountainsides on arrival;
red, gold, citrus beds of fallen leaves a week later. They were founded
in the 14th and 15th centuries and expanded in the 18th and 19th
centuries. Both sites were selected to nestle below forested mountains
and face flowing rivers with nearby fields of crops. The pattern of
their tile-roofed noble houses and thatch-roofed commoners' houses
reflects their Confucian clan structure.

The separation of places for spiritual growth and learning (head
in the air) from areas for agriculture and living (feet on the ground)
is apparent in the secluded academies on sites of scholastic retreat
beside mountain streams. Long, open pavilions bring students close
to nature and encourage ardent debate and the writing of poetry.
Libraries house treasures, and a quiet walled shrine stands behind in
its grove of crepe myrtles. Ancestor rituals, communal games, masked
plays and poetry permeate village life and lift morale at times of
misfortune.

So what in that familiar scene could be evoked for a villager with
dementia? Perhaps the sounds of water, or poetry read in language,
the sight and scent of myrtle or mountain pine, an ancient tree
representing wisdom, autumn colours, a small shrine, a step outside
to see the night sky once more? We would have to ask.

The migrant

Migrants leave behind the physical settings and communities that
underpinned their cultural identities and enter new environments
that may be hard to adjust to. Their experiences can, perhaps, act

as useful metaphors for those felt by people with dementia who are being cared for in unfamiliar places.

Australia is now a truly multicultural society and, in 2001, 23 per cent of the New South Wales population had been born overseas. In response, that year, the State National Parks & Wildlife Service set out to study the meaning and function of national parks for different ethnic communities. Although the State's recent migrants have tended to settle in urban areas, the study considered their perceptions of, and responses to, outdoor public spaces – both physically (feet on the ground) and in 'thoughts and dreams' (head in the air).

The first study discussed these questions with members of Sydney's Macedonian community. Attitudes stemmed from both the traditions of Macedonian life itself and from experiences gained as migrants growing up, or growing old, in Sydney. Early Macedonian immigrants had moved from rural villages to urban Australia and to a very different industrialised working life. Clinging together in a cohesive community was one way of ensuring some continuity in a world where everything had changed. So, they would meet en masse for picnics in parklands – where they could 'speak their own language, drink their grappa, sing and dance without ridicule'.

Traditional food of pork, sausage and cooked capsicum was well suited to the Australian barbecue. Newcomers could meet and be welcomed by others. Many of those interviewed had experienced profound problems in orienting themselves in Australia initially, and the gradual familiarity of particular parks where friends and families met had helped towards a sense of belonging. The ability to eat familiar food outdoors and to mix with friends was what mattered, rather than particulars of the natural setting, plants or wildlife.

The second study interviewed members of Sydney's Vietnamese community – both refugees and migrants. The sense of overwhelming space in the Australian bush was a constant theme. Also, the Australian concept of national parks, with land deliberately set aside for natural rather than human purposes, was astonishing – the waste was hard to comprehend. Sydney streets were sadly empty of people – big houses, closed front doors and no jostle. Domestic gardens planted with flowers and lawns rather than vegetables were similarly extraordinary – and then, in the national parks, the 'trees without a purpose, only for shade':

It's a harsh land of space and freedom.

(Nhung, 35 years)

The Vietnamese landscape is viewed as more intimate, knowable, adapted and crowded and the Australian bush as wild, unknowable, empty and potentially frightening. However, the spaciousness also signifies a sense of freedom and openness that is seen as a fine aspect of Australian culture. As with the Macedonians, the social activities undertaken in parks are crucially important to the Vietnamese, but with more mingling with other communities for picnics or barbecues. The report identifies a gradual exchange of ideas between locals and newcomers where 'new perceptions about nature are taken up and old ones discarded'.

So?

What do the reactions of these two ethnic communities to a weirdly unfamiliar landscape suggest for the care of displaced people with dementia? Perhaps that, with a generous sky above, familiar tastes and cooking smells and the sounds of people speaking a known language can help to ease away the strangeness, until the new surroundings themselves gradually become known – and safe.

This conclusion is not so different from that of the probable feelings of the inhabitants of the three described World Heritage landscapes. What is the world of the five senses that they have learnt, in earlier lives, to move through and enjoy?

Feet on the ground, habitual tasks – in surroundings with familiar sights, sounds, textures, tastes and smells. Head in the air, dreaming and recognising with joy familiar patterns of thought, cultural stories, music and songs. How much of this can we offer in a new setting?

Conclusion

How Do We Make Outside Spaces Familiar and Life-Affirming?

MARY MARSHALL AND JANE GILLIARD

We do appreciate that our book sets a real challenge to the current provision of 'gardens' in care homes, hospitals, day centres and housing. Making outside spaces familiar and life-affirming to a group of people with a host of different backgrounds is not an easy task. This is precisely true of inside spaces too. It is not difficult to make individual rooms familiar by using familiar décor, furniture and objects, but it is very challenging to make communal areas such as lounges equally familiar to everyone who lives there. But it is important to try if we want people to feel comfortable. As we said at the start, our aim is to get people with dementia outside to benefit their physical and mental health, and if an unfamiliar space is the deterrent then this needs to be energetically addressed.

The first step on this journey towards making outside spaces more familiar is to change our language. We need to talk about 'outside spaces' or 'outdoor spaces' rather than 'gardens'. If we use the term 'gardens', we immediately begin to have preconceptions about what we are trying to provide. Using a much more general term enables us to start thinking about what we should put in these spaces and frees us up to be much more responsive to the backgrounds of those people with dementia who will use it.

This leads onto the second and perhaps most crucial step, which is knowing about the backgrounds of the people with dementia who will be using the space. We know that people with dementia are often living in the past, although which years of the past vary from person to person and time to time. For some it is their early adulthood, for some their adolescence and for many their childhood. It seems to us that nature and childhood have a particular resonance. For example, Jane recently found a school report from the school her mother attended when she was about five years old and noted that nature studies was among the most important subjects, alongside reading, scripture and sums. There are few remarks on the report, except for a note that she was 'very good' at nature studies! We hope this book has demonstrated the importance of those vivid childhood memories of nature and outside space; and how diverse these memories are.

We believe that asking about memories of nature and outside spaces should be part of the initial information collected, in the same way as information is collected about hobbies, family, illnesses and so on. It is also crucial to ask about childhood and where this took place, since a lot of these history sections in case files are limited to adulthood: marriage, children, jobs. It is not just the place but the activities that are important. Recently a group of care staff talked about their childhood memories. Most of them were urban Scots; the women talked about helping their mothers hang out the washing, the men talked about playing football on any space available. It should also be borne in mind that some places have a deep significance for some people because their families have an association with them over many generations. Thus, for example, many Scots will feel that lochs and glens are part of their genetic make-up even if they have lived most of their lives in the cities. This affinity with particular locations that are important to families through the generations can be expressed as a strong feeling for 'ancestors' and where they are, which is the terminology used in some cultures.

The sort of questions that might form part of a history-taking might be:

- Where did Mrs A spend her childhood?
- Can you tell me what sort of place it was?
- Do you know what she did when she was outside?
- Does she have any special feelings for some sorts of outside areas or outside activities?
- Are there other aspects of outside which were important in her life as a young adult?

- Are there aspects of outside spaces which she might find repellent or frightening for some reason?

Person-centred care is now well established in dementia care, and fundamental to this is a knowledge of people's backgrounds and histories. We are simply suggesting that there is a part of people's histories that can be neglected but which is really important if we are to ensure that people with dementia use outside spaces happily. We need to bear in mind that we can bring the outside in, provide a view to outside or wheel a bed outside (as long as wide doors have been provided), so this does not only apply to those who are fit enough to take themselves outside. We also need to hold onto a principle of person-centred care which is about stimulating, challenging and helping people reach their full potential so new experiences of outside can be much appreciated by some people sometimes. People with dementia do not always want to be prisoners of their past all the time.

Once we are alerted to the histories of those in our care, or for whom we are designing outside spaces, our awareness of the diversity of this experience should be well reinforced. Any setting will have a mixture of people from city centre, suburban and rural/coastal backgrounds, even if not from other countries. However, as populations move more and more between countries, there will be more and more people ageing in a different country from their childhood and the extent of diverse experiences will be more apparent. So awareness of diversity is the third step.

The fourth step is building this awareness and this dimension of person-centred care into the core thinking of any establishment or design. The commitment to providing culturally appropriate outside space needs to be 'built into the bricks' in a sense rather than just aspired to. Thus we would hope to see it expressed in brochures, statements of principles, mission statements and so on. We would hope it would be part of guidance on history-taking and of training sessions. We then would expect it to be translated into care plans so that every individual care plan had a section on what sort of culturally appropriate activity was planned. This may be about outings if the need is for fields, hills or the sea, as it would be for the people Gillean Maclean mentions, but for many it is about what activities are provided on the spot. Of course, in most cases this will require a suitable outside space – which brings us to the fifth step: the design of the actual spaces.

Unless the group living in a building are truly homogenous in their past experience, the best approach to designing outside spaces may be to think about providing outside 'rooms'. (There is a long British tradition here led by Gertrude Jekyll, a garden designer of the early twentieth century.) By thinking of the outside space as rooms, different spaces can have a very different character. Thus for people who were born in the middle of a city in the North East of England, as in Karen Franks and Kate Andrews' chapter, we might think about an outside space that was more like a backyard and another which was more like a public park. For those who come from a rural area like Beth Britton's father, we may need to think about some animals for him to worry about and care for. In some care homes with many Catholic residents, a grotto is provided where people can go to do their rosary, which is a very familiar and culturally appropriate use of an outside space. A care home in a coastal area of the UK provides a washing line, not for the women but for men who have been seafarers and have always washed their own socks. Really understanding the past of people with dementia and providing meaningful spaces and activities can challenge some assumptions!

Different kinds of spaces is one requirement; another is the objects that are in the spaces to stimulate memories. For Sidsel Bjørneby's Norwegian residents, we may need to provide an old boat or some farming equipment, for example. This enables family, staff and residents to reminisce and to feel there are some connections to a more familiar life.

We will make no attempt here to describe how to design outside spaces for people with dementia which are accessible and safe, since there are books with this purpose (e.g. Pollock and Marshall 2012). We want instead to stress that outside spaces can contain different areas with different characters and activities. 'Sensory gardens' is a popular term and concept in the UK, but these are only appropriate for a minority. There may needs to be an area of conventional, fragrant garden plants, but there also need to be areas which are quite different and more familiar to those who never had a conventional garden. We may need to stress that outside spaces can be for groups or can be places to be on your own. Clearly, some of the minority groups in

Australia mentioned in Joan Domicelj's chapter will appreciate an area where they can have picnics with large family groups; other people will need familiar spaces to be alone with memories.

The fifth step again follows, which is to make the point that some experiences are universal – the sky, the weather, the seasons – and it is crucially important to people with dementia from any culture that they have the opportunity to experience them. The memories they trigger will be different, but they will inevitably be deep and individually meaningful. As we said at the start, everybody needs to go outside.

And finally the staff. Staff, too, have very different histories and memories. They, too, need outside spaces that make them feel comfortable, that awaken their basic humanity, that calm them, that make them feel valued and so on. Staff, too, need quiet, vitamin D and exercise. A staff member from southern Africa, for example, may want to sit under a tree even if the climate is different from their childhood, and to reflect on the area they came from. If we meet the needs of staff in respect of what is meaningful for them, it is much easier to demonstrate how important this can be for the people in their care. It is easy to think that people with dementia whose most familiar kind of contact with nature may not be easy to provide in a standard outside space then experience double jeopardy by being cared for by staff who themselves come from other parts of the world. However, in reality there may be more in common between a southern African care worker who comes from a rural area and a British resident who comes from a rural area than with a young British care worker who has always lived in the city centre – and of course the other way round.

We want to conclude by stressing that this is a very new approach to outside areas, where there is very little literature or guidance. We hope that this book generates lots of new ideas and approaches which will then be shared so that we can all benefit. And, more crucially, so that we can all learn how to make more outside spaces familiar and life-affirming to people with dementia.

References and Further Reading

Introduction

Care Commission and Mental Welfare Commission (2009) *Remember, I'm Still Me.* Edinburgh: Mental Welfare Commission. Available at www.mwcscot.org.uk, accessed on 3 December 2013.

Department of Health (2009) *Living Well with Dementia: A National Dementia Strategy.* Available at www.gov.uk/government/publications/living-well-with-dementia-a-national-dementia-strategy, accessed on 3 December 2013.

Department of Health (2010) *Quality Outcomes for People with Dementia: Building on the Work of the National Dementia Strategy.* Available at www.gov.uk/government/publications/quality-outcomes-for-people-with-dementia-building-on-the-work-of-the-national-dementia-strategy, accessed on 3 December 2013.

Gibson, F. (2011) *Reminiscence and Life Story Work* (4th edition). London: Jessica Kingsley Publishers.

Gilliard, J., and Marshall, M. (2012) *Transforming the Quality of Life for People with Dementia through Contact with the Natural World.* London: Jessica Kingsley Publishers.

Killick, J. (2008) *Dementia Diary: Poems and Prose.* London: Hawker Publications.

Killick, J. (ed.) (2010) *The Elephant in the Room: Poems by People with Memory Loss in Cmabridgeshire.* Cambridge: Cambridgeshire County Council.

Larson, E.B., Wang, L., Bowen, J.D., McCormick, W.C., *et al.* (2006) 'Exercise is associated with reduced risk for incident dementia among persons 65 years of age and older.' *Annals of Internal Medicine 144*, 73–81.

Lloyd-Yeates, T. (2013) 'Working one-to-one with iPads.' *Journal of Dementia Care 21*, 2, 16.

Louv, R. (2011) *The Nature Principle.* Chapel Hill, NC: Algonquin Books.

McLeod, W.T. (ed.) (1987) *The Collins Dictionary and Thesaurus in One Volume.* London: Collins.

McNair, D., Cunningham, C., Pollock, R., and McGuire, B. (2013) *Light and Lighting Design for People with Dementia.* Stirling: Dementia Services Development Centre.

Sampson, E.L., Lanchard, R.B., Jones, L., Tookman, A., and King, M. (2009) 'Dementia in the acute hospital: prospective cohort study of prevalence and mortality.' *British Journal of Psychiatry 195*, 61–66.

Scottish Government (2011) *Scotland's National Dementia Strategy 2010 – 2013.*

Ulrich, R.S. (2001) 'Effects of Healthcare Design on Medical Outcomes.' In A. Diani (ed.) *Design and Health: Proceedings of the Second International Conference on Health and Design.* Stockholm: Svensk Byggtjanst.

Welsh Assembly Government and Alzheimer's Society (2011) *National Dementia Vision for Wales.*

Chapter 5

Alzheimer's Society (2009) *Counting the Cost.* London: Alzheimer's Society.

Davis, S., Fleming, R., and Marshall, M. (2009) 'Environments that Enhance Dementia Care: Issues and Challenges.' In R. Nay and S. Garratt (eds) *Older People: Issues and Innovation in Care* (3rd edition). Chatswood, NSW, Australia: Elsevier.

Department of Health (2001) *The National Service Framework for Older People.* London: Department of Health.

Nightingale, F. (1859) *Notes on Nursing: What it Is, and What it Is Not.* London: Harrison & Sons.

Ulrich, R.S. (1984) 'View through a window may influence recovery from surgery.' *Science 224,* 4647, 420–421.

Waller, S., Masterson, A., and Finn, H. (2013) *Developing Supportive Design for People with Dementia.* London: King's Fund.

Useful website
www.kingsfund.org.uk/dementia

Chapter 8

Absolon, K.E. (Minogiizhigokwe) (2011) *Kaandossiwin: How We Come to Know.* Halifax, NS: Fernwood Publishing.

Annerstedt, M., and Wahrbourg, P. (2011) 'Nature-assisted therapy: systematic review of controlled and observational studies.' *Scandinavian Journal of Public Health 39,* 371–388.

Butler, R., Dwosh, E., Beattie, B.L., Guimond, C., *et al.* (2011) 'Genetic counseling for early-onset familial Alzheimer disease in large Aboriginal kindred from a remote community in British Columbia: unique challenges and possible solutions.' *Journal of Genetics Counselling 20,* 136–142.

Henderson, N.J. (2012, July) *Dementia: The Embodiment of Oppression.* Colloquium presentation at the Centre for Research on Personhood in Dementia, UBC, Vancouver, BC.

Hulko, W., Camille, E., Antifeau, E., Arnouse, M., Bachynski, N., and Taylor, D. (2010) 'Views of First Nation Elders on memory loss and memory care in later life.' *Journal of Cross Cultural Gerontology 25,* 317–342.

Jacklin, K., and Warry, W. (2012) 'Decolonizing First Nations Health.' In J.C. Kulig and M.N. Williams (eds) *Health in Rural Canada.* Vancouver, BC: UBC Press.

Mapes, N. (2011) *Wandering in the Woods: A Visit Woods Pilot Project July 2011.* Essex, UK: Dementia Adventure.

Chapter 9

Gaumnitz, G. (compiler) (2009) *Getting Old.* Spring Valley: Mercury Press.

Shepherd, A.P. (1991) *Rudolf Steiner – Scientist of the Invisible.* Edinburgh: Floris.

Further reading

Baum, J. (2003) *When Death Enters Life*. Edinburgh: Floris.

Camps, A., Hagenhoff, B., and van der Star, A. (2008) *Anthroposophical Care for the Elderly*. Edinburgh: Floris.

Lewis, J. (2010) *Healthy Body, Healthy Brain – Alzheimer's and Dementia Prevention and Care*. Edinburgh: Floris.

Therkleson, T. (2010) 'Ginger compress therapy for adults with osteoarthritis.' *Journal of Advanced Nursing 66*, 10, 2225–2233.

Van Bentheim, T. (2006) *Home Nursing for Carers*. Edinburgh: Floris.

Wilkinson, R. (2001) *Rudolf Steiner – An Introduction to his Spiritual World-view, Anthroposophy*. Forest Row, East Sussex: Temple Lodge.

Available on DVD

Stedall, J. (2012) *The Challenge of Rudolf Steiner*, a documentary film. Nailsworth, Gloucestershire: Cupola Productions.

Chapter 10

Care Commission and Mental Welfare Commission (2009) *Remember, I'm Still Me*. Edinburgh: Mental Welfare Commission. Available at www.mwcscot.org.uk, accessed on 3 December 2013.

Conrad, P. (1987) 'The experience of illness: recent and new directions.' *Research in the Sociology of Health Care 6*, 1–31.

Gilliard, J., and Marshall, M. (eds) (2011) *Transforming the Quality of Life for People with Dementia through Contact with the Natural World*. London: Jessica Kingsley Publishers.

Pollock, A., and Marshall, M. (2012) *Designing Outside Spaces for People with Dementia*. Stirling: University of Stirling.

Smith, J.A., and Osborn, M. (2003) 'Interpretative Phenomenological Analysis.' In J. Smith (ed.) *Qualitative Psychology: A Practical Guide to Research Methods*. London: Sage.

Chapter 12

Louv, R. (2005) *Last Child in the Woods: Saving Our Children from Nature-Deficit Disorder*. Chapel Hill, NC: Algonquin Books.

Republic of Korea (2008) *The Nomination of Historic Villages of Korea: Hahoe and Yangdong*, pp.51–54.

Further reading

Aboriginal and Torres Strait Islander Ageing Committee (2010) *Growing Old in Aboriginal Communities – Linking Services and Research*. Report of the 2nd National Workshop of the Australian Association of Gerontology, Darwin, 2010.

Cultural Diversity and Heritage. International Symposium in Commemoration of the 50th Anniversary of Japanese Law for Protection of Cultural Properties, Tokyo, 2000.

Domicelj, J. (2011) 'On the World Heritage List: the Hanoe and Yangdong Villages of Korea.' *TAASA Review*, the Journal of the Asian Arts Society of Australia, September 2011.

Domicelj, J., and Marshall, D. (1994) *Diversity, Place and the Ethics of Conservation.* Canberra: Australian Heritage Commission.

Gammage, W. (2012) *The Biggest Estate on Earth – How Aborigines Made Australia.* Crows Nest, NSW: Allen & Unwin.

Hobhouse, P. (2002) *The Story of Gardening.* New York: Dorling Kindersley.

Ikeda, M. (1993) *Ancient Fantasies – The Ceramic Works of Masuo Ikeda.* Japan.

Martin, H. (2002) *The Sheltering Desert* (new edition). Hamburg: Two Books. (First English edition by William Kimber 1957.)

Moss, S. (2012) *Natural Childhood.* London: National Trust.

Pollock, A., and Marshall, M. (2012) *Designing Outdoor Spaces for People with Dementia.* Stirling: University of Stirling.

Rose, D.B. (1996) *Nourishing Terrains – Australian Aboriginal Views of Landscape and Wilderness.* Canberra: Australian Heritage Commission.

Saito, H. (ed.) (1996) *World Heritage: the Historic Villages of Shirakawa-go and Gokayama – Traditional Houses in the Gassho Style.* Committee for the Commemoration of the Inscription, Japan.

Taylor, K., and Lennon, J. (eds) (2012) *Managing Cultural Landscapes.* London: Routledge.

Thomas, M. (2001) *A Multicultural Landscape – National Parks and the Macedonian Experience.* Sydney: NSW National Parks & Wildlife Service.

Thomas, M. (2002) *Moving Landscapes – National Parks and the Vietnamese Experience.* Sydney: NSW National Parks & Wildlife Service.

Timms, P. (1999) *The Nature of Gardens.* St Leonards, NSW: Allen & Unwin.

Conclusion

Pollock, A., and Marshall, M. (2012) *Designing Outside Spaces for People with Dementia.* Stirling: University of Stirling.

About the Editors

Jane Gilliard is a social worker who has worked in dementia care, especially concerning design for people with dementia, for over 25 years. She established Dementia Voice, the dementia services development centre for Southwest England, and was its director from 1997 to 2005; she chaired the National Network of Dementia Services Development Centres; was a member of the National Institute for Clinical Excellence (NICE)/Social Care Institute for Excellence (SCIE) Guideline Development Group; and sat on the Working Group that developed the National Dementia Strategy for England.

Mary Marshall is a social worker who has worked with and for older people for most of her professional career. She was the director of the Dementia Services Development Centre at the University of Stirling from 1989 until she retired in 2005. She now writes and lectures on dementia care. She chaired the steering group for the new dementia standards in Scotland.

About the Authors

Kate Andrews is an NHS counselling psychologist in Gateshead, UK, working with older adults, and has a special interest in challenging behaviour and dementia. Her interests include the importance of attachment across the lifespan and its application in people with dementia.

Sidsel Bjørneby was born in Lillehammer, Norway, in 1939. She is a retired occupational therapist and senior lecturer who has in the last 20 years been involved in a number of European and Norwegian research and development projects about adapting products, systems and environments to people with dementia. Presently she is associated with the Oslo Geriatric Resource Centre.

Beth Britton is a dementia campaigner and care consultant, writer and blogger. Her father had vascular dementia for approximately the last 19 years of his life. She aims to provide support and advice to those faced with similar situations, inform and educate care professionals and the wider population, promote debate and create improvements in dementia care.

Joan Domicelj, AM, is an Australian architect, planner and mediator. She has been named one of the '60 Women Contributing to the 60 Years of UNESCO', in the fields of cultural diversity and heritage.

Karen Franks is an NHS consultant in old-age psychiatry in Gateshead, UK. Her interests include improving care for those in 24-hour care settings and trying to maintain links between all those with an interest in good-quality dementia care in an increasingly fragmented health and social care system.

Wendy Hulko is an associate professor in the School of Social Work and Human Service at Thompson Rivers University in Kamloops, BC, and a researcher with the Centre for Research on Personhood in Dementia at the University of British Columbia. Wendy holds a BA degree in Sociology and Spanish, a Masters in Social Work and a PhD in Sociology and Social Policy. She has worked in the field of ageing since 1993. Since 2007 Wendy has been researching First Nation views on memory loss in later life and culturally safe dementia care in collaboration with Secwepemc Nation Elders and decision-makers from the local health authority.

Yutaka Inoue, D. of Eng. is Professor of Real Estate Sciences, Meikai University, Japan, where he has been teaching and undertaking research on architecture and related fields since 1995. He has authored several books including the translation of *Design for Dementia* (co-edited by Mary Marshall) and a book on care homes in Northern European countries.

Judith Jones has been living and working in Camphill communities since 1973, initially as a teacher and houseparent for children with special needs. Later she trained as a nurse and in 2002 joined Simeon Care for the Elderly. Judith has recently retired and still lives on the Simeon site.

John Killick has been Poet Mentor for the dementia project at the Courtyard Centre for the Arts in Hereford and writer in residence for Alzheimer Scotland since 1993. He has worked as a writer with people with dementia for over 20 years, and has published 11 books on the subject; his latest is Dementia Positive (Luath Press 2013).

Gillean Maclean, a former nurse, is now a parish minister of the Church of Scotland living and working in Aberdeenshire. Much of her ministry has been in rural settings. She has always been interested in the quality of care provided for those in our community who are now of mature years. This interest became personal when her mother was diagnosed with dementia. Gillean was involved for a time in providing services of worship for those with dementia and their carers and continues to seek ways to minister effectively to people who are unable to attend services for a variety of reasons both in residential care settings and at home.

Neil Mapes is the founder and director of Dementia Adventure CIC. He is a Clore Social Fellow and in 2012 successfully completed the inaugural Clore Social Leadership Programme. Neil was recently selected by an expert panel of judges at NESTA and the *Observer* newspaper as one of 'Britain's New Radicals' – 50 people and organisations changing Britain for the better. Neil has a background in clinical psychology and dementia advocacy and also has experience of leading adventure travel holidays in Europe, Asia Minor and South America.

Abigail Masterson, MPa, MN, BSc, RGN, PGCEA, FRSA, has been supporting the evaluation of the Enhancing the Healing Environment (EHE) projects focused on dementia. She is a nurse with clinical expertise in older people's services, and has extensive experience in evaluating service and practice developments both in the UK and internationally.

James McKillop, MBE, is living with dementia. He is now 72. He lives at home with his wife and younger son and is involved in various groups which deal with people with learning difficulties. Until recently, he was out nearly every day at activities, conferences, etc. However, physical ill health has now curtailed his outings. Luckily, the dementia movement marches on. James recently received an honorary doctorate at the University of Strathclyde.

Margaret-Anne Tibbs grew up and qualified as a social worker in South Africa. On coming to the UK she worked as a social worker and then a trainer in social care for 25 years, where she had extensive involvement with staff from overseas. She has many close friends from southern Africa.

Sarah Waller, CBE, RGN, FRSA, is the Programme Director for The King's Fund's Enhancing the Healing Environment (EHE) programme. She joined The King's Fund in 2000 to develop the programme having had a long career working at all levels in the NHS both in nursing and human resource management.

Subject Index

Author Index

Transforming the Quality of Life for People with Dementia through Contact with the Natural World

Fresh Air on My Face

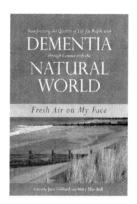

Edited by Jane Gilliard and Mary Marshall

Paperback: £16.99/$26.95
ISBN: 978 1 84905 267 2
160 pages

This important book simply but persuasively demonstrates why we should provide opportunities for people with dementia to experience the great outdoors. It also gives a voice to people with dementia who have felt the benefit of getting closer to nature. The contributors explore many different ways in which people with dementia can experience and interact with nature through pursuits such as farming, gardening and walking, and the book includes a chapter on the therapeutic, life-enhancing effects of activities with animals.

The book includes descriptions of projects and initiatives from around the world that have revolutionised the everyday experience of people with dementia, and made a real difference to their quality of life. Illustrated with photographs amply demonstrating the power of nature to lift the spirits and enrich life, the book will be an inspiring guide for relatives, carers and professionals who want to help people with dementia lead a richer life, experience nature fully and enjoy its many accompanying benefits.

Jane Gilliard is a social worker who has worked in dementia care for over 25 years. She established Dementia Voice, the dementia services development centre for South West England, and was its director from 1997 to 2005. Jane chaired the national network of Dementia Services Development Centres, was a member of the NICE/SCIE Guideline Development Group, and also sat on the Working Group that developed the National Dementia Strategy for England. **Mary Marshall** is a social worker who has worked with and for older people for most of her professional career. She was the director of the Dementia Services Development Centre at the University of Stirling from 1989 until she retired in 2005, and now writes and lectures in dementia care. Mary chaired the steering group for the new dementia standards in Scotland.

Playfulness and Dementia
A Practice Guide

John Killick

Bradford Dementia Group Good
Practice Guides series

Paperback: £16.99/$27.95
ISBN: 978 1 84905 223 8
120 pages

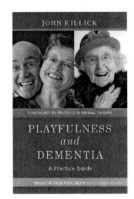

Establishing playfulness as an essential
component of dementia care, this positive and
uplifting book will be key in changing attitudes
and providing ideas for new and valuable ways of interacting and being
with individuals with the condition.

John Killick explores the nature of playfulness and the many ways
in which it can enrich the lives of people with dementia, including as
a means of maintaining relationships and communication, supporting
communication and generally lifting the spirits. Specific approaches
already in existence are described, including improvised drama,
clowning and laughter yoga, and a chapter on a playful approach to
art and craft activities is also included. Personal accounts of playfulness
by individuals with dementia, relatives and an actor with a decade's
experience of using playful approaches with people with dementia offer
rich first-hand insights into its transformative potential. Throughout
the book, the importance of spontaneity and of being with the person
with dementia in the present moment is emphasised, and the reader
is encouraged to develop a playful mindset. A selection of colour
photographs amply demonstrate playful approaches in action.

Offering a fresh and perhaps unexpected perspective, this book is
essential reading for dementia care practitioners and managers, activity
coordinators, therapists, people with dementia and their relatives, and
anyone else concerned with the wellbeing of those with the condition.

John Killick has worked with people with dementia for over 16 years, in care homes,
day centres, hospital wards and in their own homes. He is known internationally for
his pioneering poetry work, but has also explored the possibilities of using a variety of
other art forms to enhance communication. He is passionately committed to providing
opportunities for people with dementia everywhere to take part in creative activities,
and has lectured, written, broadcast and run training sessions on the subject in a number
of different countries. He is currently Writer in Residence for Alzheimer Scotland and
runs an improvised drama group for the Scottish Dementia Working Group. He is the
co-author of *Creativity and Communication in Persons with Dementia*, also published by JKP.

Personalisation and Dementia
A Guide for Person-Centred Practice

Helen Sanderson and Gill Bailey

Paperback: £25.00/$39.95
ISBN: 978 1 84905 379 2
192 pages

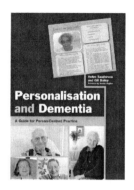

Personalisation builds on person-centred care to focus on how people with dementia can have more choice and control over decisions affecting them, and be supported to be part of their communities.

This practical guide explains how to deliver personalised services and support for people with dementia through simple, evidence-based person-centred practices. The authors clearly explain personalisation and current person-centred thinking and practice, providing many vivid examples of how it has been achieved in community as well as residential care settings. They guide the reader through using a range of person-centred practices. Strategies for ensuring a good match between the person with dementia and the staff and volunteers supporting them are also described. In the final chapter, the reader is introduced to Progress for Providers, a photocopiable tool for tracking progress in delivering appropriate personalised support for people with dementia living in care homes.

This is essential reading for dementia care practitioners and managers, as well as social and health care workers, community workers and students.

Helen Sanderson is CEO of Helen Sanderson Associates (HSA) and Director Emeritus of the International Community for Person-Centred Practices. She has been closely involved in the development of person-centred thinking and planning in the UK over the last fifteen years. She is the author of *A Practical Guide to Delivering Personalisation* and *Creating Person-Centred Organisations*, both published by JKP. HSA's partnership with Borough Care Ltd and Stockport Council were runners up in the National Dementia Awards 2012 in the innovation category. **Gill Bailey** trained initially as a nurse and has worked with a range of providers and commissioning units across adult health and social care for over twenty-five years, and in the last ten years this has focussed on supporting people living with dementia. She is a Dementia Care Mapper, has a diploma in Dementia Studies and is studying for a master's degree in this area. She is currently working with providers to introduce Individual Service funds in residential and homecare services for people living with dementia.

Risk Assessment and Management for Living Well with Dementia

Charlotte L. Clarke, Heather Wilkinson, John Keady and Catherine E. Gibb

Bradford Dementia Group Good Practice Guides series

Paperback: £16.99/$32.95
ISBN: 978 1 84905 005 0
128 pages

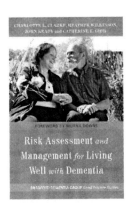

Winner in the Health and Social Care category at the 2012 British Medical Association Book Awards

Risk is central to professional practice, assessment and decision-making in dementia care. Yet theories of risk are often complex and difficult to translate into everyday practice.

This book outlines some of the key issues in risk perception, assessment and management in dementia care in a way that is both practical and accessible to a wide range of practitioners. It develops an approach to risk that promotes choice for people with dementia whilst also acknowledging the complex challenges care providers face. The authors provide an overview of the legislative framework currently in place, and of the ethical dilemmas which may emerge in practice. Frameworks for informed and balanced decision-making are offered, and the importance of including the person with dementia, their family, and care providers in decision-making is emphasised. Throughout the book, case studies are used to illustrate effective negotiation and practical solutions to risk dilemmas in practice.

This book highlights principles of good practice for managing risk in dementia care, and presents a rounded approach that will help practitioners negotiate some of the complex issues this entails.

Charlotte L. Clarke is Professor of Nursing Practice Development Research and Associate Dean at Northumbria University. **Heather Wilkinson** is Co-Director of the Centre for Research on Families and Relationships and Research Director for the School of Health in Social Science at the University of Edinburgh. **John Keady** is Professor of Older People's Mental Health Nursing at the University of Manchester and Greater Manchester West Mental Health NHS Foundation Trust. **Catherine E. Gibb** is a Senior Lecturer at Northumbria University.

The Pool Activity Level (PAL) Instrument for Occupational Profiling
A Practical Resource for Carers of People with Cognitive Impairment

4th edition

Jackie Pool

Bradford Dementia Group Good Practice Guides series

Paperback: £26.99/$45.00
ISBN: 978 1 84905 221 4
224 pages

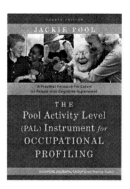

The Pool Activity Level (PAL) Instrument is widely used as the framework for providing activity-based care for people with cognitive impairments, including dementia. The Instrument is recommended for daily living skills training and activity planning in the National Institute for Clinical Excellence Clinical Guidelines for Dementia (NICE 2006), and has been proven valid and reliable by a recent research study. It is an essential resource for any practitioner or carer wanting to provide fulfilling occupation for clients with cognitive impairments.

This fourth edition of *The Pool Activity Level (PAL) Instrument for Occupational Profiling* includes a new section on using the PAL Checklist to carry out sensory interventions, together with the photocopiable Instrument itself in a new easy-to-use format, and plans that help to match users' abilities to activities. It includes the latest research on the use of the PAL Instrument in a range of settings, and new case studies, as well as information about how a new online PAL tool complements and supports the book. The book also contains suggestions for activities, together with information on obtaining the necessary resources and guidance for carrying out the activities with individuals of different ability levels, as revealed by the PAL Checklist.

Jackie Pool is an Occupational Therapist specialising in the development and provision of programmes and materials for leadership and workforce development in dementia care. She sat on the National Dementia Strategy Reference Group and was commissioned by Skills for Care to write the QCF dementia units for the national health and social care qualifications. She has published extensively and speaks at many conferences in the field of dementia care. Jackie's website can be found at www.jackiepoolassociates.org.

Enriched Care Planning for People with Dementia

A Good Practice Guide to Delivering Person-Centred Care

Hazel May, Paul Edwards and Dawn Brooker

Bradford Dementia Group Good
Practice Guides series

Paperback: £25.00/$49.95
ISBN: 978 1 84310 405 6
176 pages

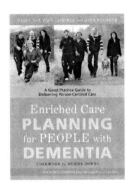

The correlation between 'disengagement' and illness in people with dementia living in long-term care settings is becoming more widely recognised, and developing and adapting front-line staff responses to the changing needs of individuals is a crucial factor in addressing this problem.

This book presents a complete practical framework for whole person assessment, care planning and review of persons with dementia or signs of dementia (including those with learning disabilities) who are in need of, or already receiving, health and/or social support. The book provides photocopiable assessment forms, guidelines for carrying out the assessment, and suggestions for tailored interventions based on the profile that emerges from the assessment process. The authors also include a clear explanation of the five theoretical components of dementia that are considered in the assessment: health, biography, personality, neurological impairment and social psychology. This good practice guide will provide a step up to the challenge of providing person-centred care as a minimum standard rather than just an ideal.

Care workers in residential settings and social workers assessing clients for their support requirements will find this an essential resource.

Hazel May is a state-registered occupational therapist with a Master's Degree in Philosophy and Health Care. She currently works for the Bradford Dementia Group as a dementia care practice development consultant and trainer based from her home in Wiltshire. **Paul Edwards** is also a dementia care practice development consultant and trainer with the Bradford Dementia Group. Paul is a mental health nurse by profession, and previously spent many years developing person-centred practice in the NHS. He lives in Leicestershire. **Professor Dawn Brooker** is the Director of the University of Worcester Association for Dementia Studies. Professionally qualified as a clinical psychologist, she has over twenty-five years' experience working to improve the quality of care for people with dementia as a clinician, as a service manager and as an academic.

CPSIA information can be obtained at www.ICGtesting.com
Printed in the USA
BVOW03s1446110714

358559BV00006BA/18/P